Physiotherap
in
Neuro-conditions

Physiotherapy in Neuro-conditions

Glady Samuel Raj
MSc PT (Bombay), MIAP, MHPC (UK)
Specialist in Neurological Physiotherapy
Principal, Padmashree Institute of Physiotherapy
Bangalore

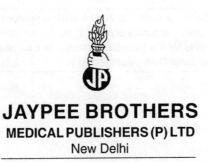

JAYPEE BROTHERS
MEDICAL PUBLISHERS (P) LTD
New Delhi

Published by

Jitendar P Vij

Jaypee Brothers Medical Publishers (P) Ltd

EMCA House, 23/23B Ansari Road, Daryaganj

New Delhi 110 002, India

Phones: +91-11-23272143, +91-11-23272703, +91-11-23282021, +91-11-23245672

Fax: +91-11-23276490, +91-11-23245683

e-mail: jaypee@jaypeebrothers.com

Visit our website: www.jaypeebrothers.com

Branches

- 2/B, Akruti Society, Jodhpur Gam Road Satellite
  Ahmedabad 380015, Phone: +91-79-30988717
- 202 Batavia Chambers, 8 Kumara Krupa Road
  Kumara Park East, **Bangalore** 560 001
  Phones:+91-80-22285971, +91-80-22382956, +91-80-30614073
  Tele Fax : +91-80-22281761   e-mail: jaypeemedpubbgl@eth.net
- 282 IIIrd Floor, Khaleel Shirazi Estate, Fountain Plaza
  Pantheon Road, **Chennai** 600 008
  Phones: +91-44-28262665, +91-44-28269897
  Fax: +91-44-28262331   e-mail: jpchen@eth.net
- 4-2-1067/1-3, 1st Floor, Balaji Building, Ramkote Cross Road
  Hyderabad 500 095, Phones: +91-40-55610020, +91-40-24758498
  Fax: +91-40-24758499   e-mail: jpmedpub@rediffmail.com
- 1A Indian Mirror Street, Wellington Square
  Kolkata 700 013, Phones: +91-33-22456075, +91-33-22451926
  Fax: +91-33-22456075   e-mail: jpbcal@cal.vsnl.net.in
- 106 Amit Industrial Estate, 61 Dr SS Rao Road
  Near MGM Hospital, Parel, **Mumbai** 400 012
  Phones: +91-22-24124863, +91-22-24104532, +91-22-30926896
  Fax: +91-22-24160828   e-mail: jpmedpub@bom7.vsnl.net.in
- "KAMALPUSHPA" 38, Reshimbag
  Opp. Mohota Science College, Umred Road, **Nagpur** 440 009 (MS)
  Phones: +91-712-3945220,+91-712-2704275, e-mail: jpmednagpur@rediffmail.com

Physiotherapy in Neuro-conditions

First Edition: **2006**

ISBN 81-8061-631-2

Typeset at   JPBMP typesetting unit

Printed at   Sanat Printers.

to

Late Mr T Arulmani
my father for inducing principles that guides my life.

Mrs Chellathai Arulmani
my mother for all her prayers and wishes.

Mrs Bernis
my beloved wife for her constant love and encouragement.

Mr Jerrin
my son for making my life joyful and worthy.

My teachers
for their guidance in every step of my life.

All dear physiotherapy students
for being the motivation behind this book.

Foreword

It gives me immense pleasure to write the foreword for this excellent book on neurophysiotherapy, which I have no doubt will be of great help to the undergraduate students. Neurophysiotherapy is for those who have sustained a neurological injury from a brain or incomplete spinal cord injury, stroke or a disease processes like multiple sclerosis. Neurophysiotherapy is a fast emerging specialized field in physiotherapy, 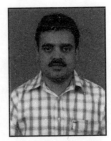 where students need reference material on this subject but sadly there are few books on neurophysiotherapy and this is the first such book by an Indian author. This book provides details on working with neurological movement disorders both adult and pediatric with a theoretical basis for clinical practice. It will enhance the physiotherapists' awareness of other aspects of client management and will provide them with a framework to develop evidence-based practice.

Prof Glady Samuel Raj has been associated with Padmashree Institute of Physiotherapy since many years. I must say as the head of the institution, he has set standards of excellence in teaching and he is also a very good therapist who gives utmost importance to the patients and their well-being. He has an authority in the field of neurophysiotherapy and responsible for the name and fame of Padmashree Institute of Physiotherapy in South-East Asia.

I do hope that Prof Glady Samuel will continue his good work and bring out many more books pertaining to the field of physiotherapy for the benefit of the student community. I admire Prof Glady Samuel for keeping the contents of the book very simple and more importantly for keeping the cost of this book within the reach of the students community.

Dr Ashwath Narayan C N
Managing Trustee
Padmashree Charitable Trust
Bangalore

Preface

It gives me immense pleasure to present my first edition of this book titled "*Physiotherapy in Neuro-conditions*" to all the physiotherapy students and professionals. This effort of mine is only a small mark of respect and passion for my profession that has given me so much during the last one decade.

Neurological physiotherapy is one of the mainstream physiotherapy branches with tremendous potential and prospect. Althoug stroke may be popular conditions in neurology, which demands constant intervention by a physiotherapist, but there are still many conditions where physiotherapy becomes very essential both as a conservative measure and after surgical intervention. If fifty percent of improvement during the treatment of a neurological conditions is through medication or surgery then the remaining fifty percent is definitely by physiotherapy.

Thus, all the common neurological conditions treated by the physiotherapists have been included in this book, which I believe will be of great use to the readers.

The book is written keeping in mind the undergraduate students of physiotherapy and hence does not focus too much upon the investigations or the differential diagnosis.

The main aim of this textbook was to present the fact of neurological physiotherapy to the students in the most simplified manner possible so that it would be easy for them to grasp its content.

The language used is very simple and the content very concise that will enable maximum information be reproduced by the students in the exam without having to put in too much effort.

I firmly believe that it is not so important to write as much as I can in a textbook but it is how much the readers have understood and can remember that matters the most. Thus, this book is written keeping in mind the same principle.

Although the book is concise, but it is definitely updated with all possible recent advances in the field of neurological physiotherapy. All suggestion and comments will be accepted by me with a warm welcome and would further motivate me during such similar venture. I sincerely hope that the readers thoroughly enjoy reading every word in the textbook that will make me feel that my effort has paid me rich dividends.

Glady Samuel Raj

Acknowledgements

First and foremost, I thank my Lord and Savior Jesus Christ without whose divine wisdom I would not have been able to complete this book.

I thank my wife, my son, my mother and all the members of my family for being a constant source of love and moral throughout my life.

I express my humble gratitude and thanks to my teachers Prof Manik Sahani, Prof Dastoor, Prof Amita Mehta, Prof Hutoxi Writer, Prof Rajeshree Sabnis, Prof Bharti Bellare, Prof Jacob, Prof Saraswati Iyer and all other senior faculty in Physiotherapy from whom I have learnt various things in professional sector.

I also express my sincere thanks to Dr Ashwath Narayana, Managing Director, Dr Vasudeva and all other members of the managing committee of Padmashree Institute of Physiotherapy for their constant support and encouragement.

I thank the following list of friends, well-wishers, and colleagues who had been instrumental in various ways that enabled me to complete this book:

Mr Timswauger, Ms Priya, Ms Sona, Ms Deepa, Ms Swathi, Ms Rajani, Mrs Anita Prem, Mr Shreethar, Mr Arun Prasad, Mr Venkatesh, Mr Dandhapani, Mr Sandeep, Mr Ratish, Prof Savita Ravindran, Prof CK Sentil Kumar, Mr Pearlson, Mr Hemant, Mr Bala Saravanan, Mr Stephen O'Brien, Mr Iftikar, Mr Ramesh, Mr Jasobant Sethi, Mr Pramod Giri, Ms Juhi Giri, Mr Sanjay Epean, Mr Dhanesh Mr Preeth Cherian, Mr Arun Maiya, Ms Bamini, Mr Amitesh Narayan, Ms Sailaxmi Ganeshan, Mr Subhash Katri, Mr Jibi Paul, Mr Karthikeyan, Mr Ram Prasad.

Special thanks to my students namely Sharmila, Latika, Farhana and Mani who had helped me in the art work of this book.

I thank all the patients who volunteered for this textbook.

Lastly, I express my sincere thanks to all those individuals who have directly or indirectly helped in this effort of mine.

Contents

Plate 1

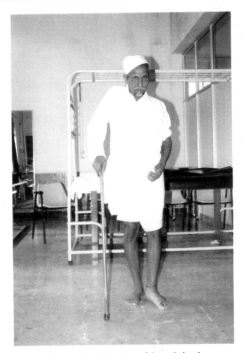

Fig. 2.2: Attitude of hemiplegic

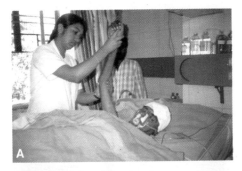

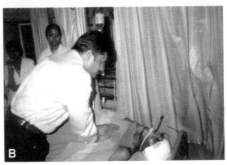

Figs 4.1A to B: Passive maneuver and chest
PT for unconscious patient

Plate 2

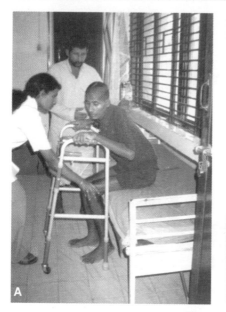
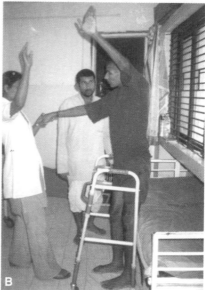
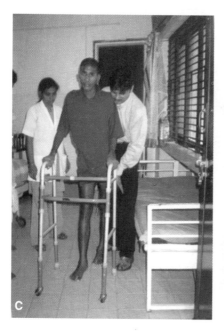
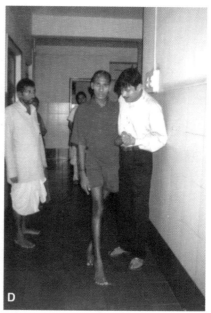

Figs 4.2A to D: Progression to walking in head injury

Plate 3

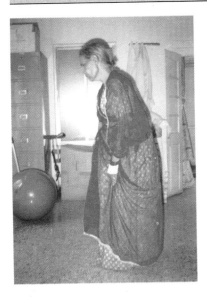

Fig. 5.2B: Posture in lateral view

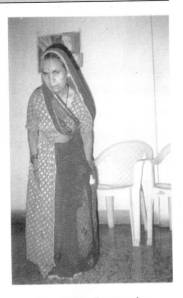

Fig. 5.3B: Posture in anterior view

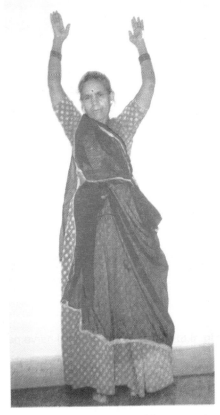

Fig. 5.5: Mobility with breathing excercises

Plate 4

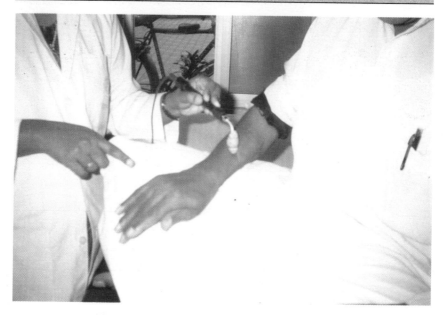

Fig. 6.5: Interrupted galvanic current stimulation

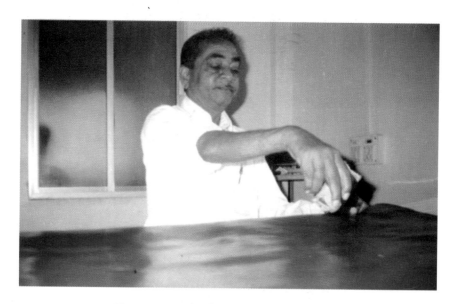

Fig. 6.6: Defective grip in radial nerve palsy

Plate 5

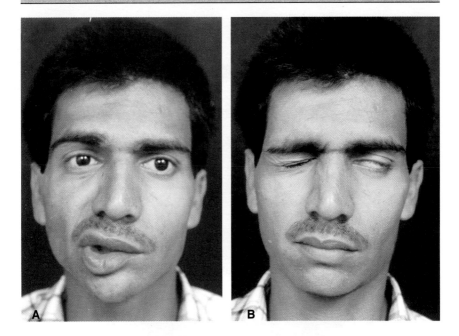

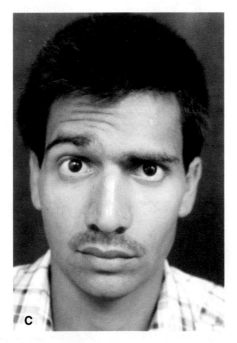

Figs 6.13A to C: Muscular imbalance in Bell's palsy

Plate 6

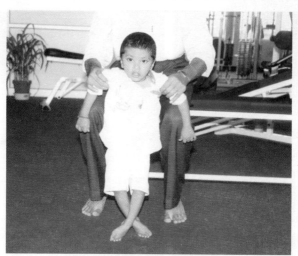

Fig. 12.1: Abnormal attitude of CP child

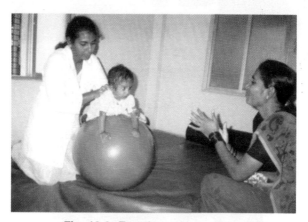

Fig. 12.2: Exercises with vestibular ball

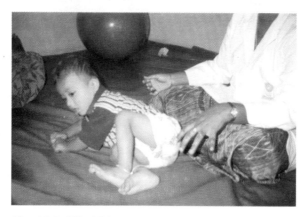

Fig. 12.3: CP child assuming sitting position after treatment

Plate 7

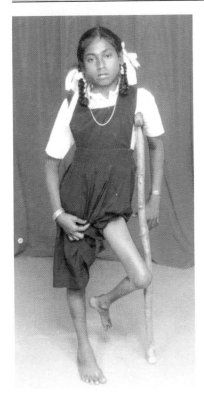

Fig. 13.1: Contracture noted in PPRP

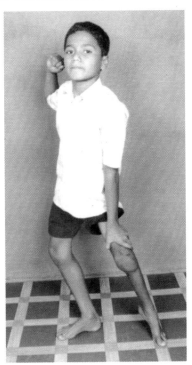

Fig. 13.2: Hand to knee gait in PPRP

1

Neurological Examination for Physiotherapist

Before beginning the actual assessment of the patient certain demographic data need to be taken which are as follows:
- Name
- Age/sex
- Address
- Occupation
- Dominance

Chief Complaint

The patient needs to be asked about his main complain that has prompted him to seek the help of the therapist. The patient should give his complains in his own simple words as completely as possible. The main concern of the patient is his level of independence in day-to-day activities and hence the chief complains are usually given as inability to eat, difficulty in dressing, difficulty in walking independently, etc. Patient is either unaware or not bothered about the physiological and pathological abnormality present in this nervous system. His complains will consists of the ultimate out comes of all the abnormality. Chief complains gives clue to the therapist as to what goal he should set for the patient and also it guides the therapist in the whole assessment. Nothing can give more pleasure to the patient than getting rid of the chief complaints. Giving the patient complete relief from his chief complains is the main aim of any intervention towards which the whole assessment gets directed.

History

A good and tactfully taken clinical history often holds key to diagnosis. A skillfully taken history with a careful analysis of the chief complaints and course of illness usually gives clue towards differential diagnosis even before the actual examination is carried out. Patience, kindness, diplomacy, friendly attitude, manner suggesting interest and compassion are some essential features that help in extracting the necessary information from the patient. While taking the history the therapist gets an opportunity to study the patient's mannerism, attitude, behavior and emotional reactions. Some patients may be either very reserved or eccentric. Eccentric patient generally siege this opportunity to communicate and may go on and on with their detailed insignificant explanation, even giving lot of importance to the doctor shopping he/she underwent. It is actually the skill of the therapist to guide the communication to what he wants and note down only those contents that is necessary for the whole assessment that will guide his to the target. The history generally is classified into different types.

Present Medical History

This should consist information about the type of onset, whether acute, subacute or chronic. Duration of the illness since the onset. Progression of the disorder—stable, condition improving, or condition deteriorating. In case of associated pain, it is necessary to find out the aggravating factor and ceasing factor. The presence of associated features like speech abnormalities, visual disturbance, bladde or bowel problem etc. should be interrogated. The various treatment taken by the patient needs to be noted. Brief note on the day-to-day function, home situation, mobility, self-care may also be taken in the history. Lastly the present state of the patient needs to be emphasized. History should eventually be related to the chief complaints of the patient.

Past History

Between past history and present history there should be time when the patient was absolutely normal. The past history could be a previous episode of the present illness (presence of TIA before the attack of stroke) or it could be a separate illness that is no way related to the present illness of the patient. Past history should be differentiated from chronic problem with acute episode or exacerbation.

Personal History

Regarding the patients habit, about risk factors, lifestyle, diet, etc.

Social History

Socioeconomic status, attitude of the family towards the patient.

Family History

Family history to rule out any hereditary predisposition should also be taken.

OBSERVATION

- *Posture and attitude:* The overall posture of the patient and the attitude of the body parts needs to be noticed.
- *Wasting:* Wasting of the muscle bulk is more pronounced in lower motor neuron in comparison to upper motor neuron. The muscles or groups of muscles that appears to be wasted on comparison with the non-affected side should be clearly specified. The distribution of wasting should be noted as it may give clue to the involved structure in lower motor neuron problem. In upper motor neuron of chronic variety the wasting seen is because of disuse.
- *Trophic changes:* These usually appear as dry scaly skin, brittleness of the nails and is suggestive of prolonged immobilization or autonomous dysfunction.
- *Involuntary movements:* Observation should be made for tremors, athetosis, chorea etc.
- *Swelling:* Swelling usually occurs due to the presence of edema and is confined to the distal parts of the extremities. It could be due to lack of mobility or it can occur as a feature of some complications like RSD.
- Certain abnormal psychological features like depression, over excitability, emotional liability, etc. can be made out on observation.

EXAMINATION

Higher Function

- *Consciousness:* Consciousness reflects the capacity of an individual state of awareness and responsiveness to his own body, as well as to the external environment. The patient may be conscious, alert, accessible and attentive, drowsy or lethargic, may show very delayed responses, in cloudy state, semicomatose or comatose, etc. Ideally for evaluation of neurological cases it is necessary to find out whether the patient is completely unconscious or semiconscious or is he completely conscious and fully aware of the things around him. The level of conscious will definitely determine the type of physical therapy treatment given to the patient.

- *Behavior:* The patient may be irritable, hostile, over anxious, resistive, shy, tense, agitated, fearful, inhibited, negative, frank, social, or friendly. The therapist should observe the patient mannerism, speech, his interest in the conversation, whether he is easily distractible, confused, absorbed, preoccupied or has decreased attention span. The patient and therapist rapport as well as understanding is necessary for a effective treatment program.

- *Memory:* Memory is achieved by means of various physiological and psychological process which extends between the perception of a stimulus and its recall or reproduction. The patient needs to be assessed for his long term memory (retrieval of information after days, months or year), short term memory (retrieval of information after several minutes or hours) and immediate memory (immediate recall or repetition of word, sentences or events). For testing long term memory one can obtain information regarding chronological events like date and place of birth, age, year when he was off the school, date of marriage, reciting nursery rhymes, alphabets, etc.

  Short-term memory may be tested by asking him about the recent meals, when he came to the hospital, with whom he came, at around what time he got up in the morning, name of the doctors attending to him, etc.

  To test the patients ability to immediately recall he may be given name, address, phone numbers and asked to recall it after 3 minutes, 15 minutes, 30 minutes or 1 hour.

- *Intelligent capacity:* Examination of the intellectual capacity of the patient is very important for the diagnostic, and prognostic point of view. Intelligent patient are generally quite sharp in relating their symptoms and grasping the exercise program designed for them which facilitates the treatment procedure. Estimation of the patient's intelligence can be made from his educational and professional level, social development, performance in the school, etc. Patient ability to do simple calculation, communication skills also shows evidence about his intellectual capacity. Certain tests like Binet-Simon test, Wechslers intelligence scale, Kuhlmann test assess a person by means of verbal tests involving information, comprehension, arithmetic, vocabulary and performance tests like picture arrangement, picture completion, block design, etc.

- *Counting and calculation:* The patient's ability to count and calculate may be evaluated by means of simple test. He may be asked to count forward or backward, count coins, may be given simple addition and subtraction. He many be asked questions like if he has three apples and five more is given to him, how many apple will he have. If a rope is 2 rupees per feet how much will fifteen feet rope cost. If ones salary is 20 rupees per day and every day he spends 10 rupees. How many days will he need to save 400 rupees. This kind of simple calculation test can be given for adult patients to find the patients ability to calculate.

- *Speech:* The patient should be tested for his ability to understand, and respond to a question in a correct manner. The clarity of speech, tone, smoothness, articulation need to be assessed.

- *Reading and writing:* The patient ability to read, his capacity to write dictated words, copy down certain text material should be tested. If a patient is not able to communicate, then his ability to understand our question can be made out by asking him to reply in writing.

- *Orientation:* The patient's orientation to time and place should be found out. He may be asked questions like what time of the day is it or where does he think he is at present. This gives adequate information to the examiner as to whether the patient is able to recognize the time and place respectively.

Cranial Nerve Examination

- *Olfactory:* This is responsible for the sensation of smell. The smell is tested by the use of non-irritating volatile oils or liquids. Each nostril is examined separately when the other is closed. The substances most commonly used are clove oil, rose water, eucalyptus oil, asafetida, coffee powder, turpentine oil, etc. The patient is asked to breathe heavily and then identify the substances. Inability to smell properly is called as *anosmia*.

- *Optic nerve:* The patient is tested for visual acuity, color vision and for visual field. Visual acuity is tested for both distant and near vision. Distance vision is checked by use of Snellen test charts. The chart is placed at a distance of 20 feet or 6 meters and the patient is asked to read it. Each eye is examined separately. Near vision can be tested by use of Jaeger's test types. It consists of paragraphs that are printed in a successively coarser type. The finest is numbered 0 and the coarser one that consists of letter that is relatively biggest is marked as 7 and the patient has to read through the whole thing.

The patient is also tested for identifying or matching colors. Some patients do have day blindness and night blindness. The most common way of testing for visual field is by using the confrontation method. In confrontation method the examiner stands with one eyelid closed in front of the patient at 2-3 feet distance who also closes his opposite eye (if examiner closes the left then the patient has to close the right). The other eye of the patient is fixed on the examiner's nose similarly the examiner fixes his eye on the patient's nose. A pencil or finger may be used as a test object. The object is moved in the visual field at an angle of 90-degree starting from the center. The patient should be able to see the object without moving the eyeball from the fixed point.

- *Ocular nerves:* As the oculomotor, trochlear and abducens nerves are responsible for the movements of the eyeball because of the link with the extraocular muscles they are termed as ocular nerves.

  The ocular movements are tested by having the patient look in the nine cardinal directions—laterally, medially, upward and laterally, upward and medially, downward and medially, downward and laterally, as well as directly upward, directly downward and finally convergence. Abnormality in the gaze can also be made out by having the patient perform a circular eye movement.

- *Trigeminal nerve:* The trigeminal nerve is a mixed nerve performing sensory and motor function. The two fibers need to be examined separately. For examining the sensory function of the nerve various exteroceptive modalities like superficial pain, thermal, light touch sensations are examined individually over the skin of the face. The cornea, conjunctiva, gums and inside of the cheeks. The motor examination consists of checking the muscle power of the masticatory muscles namely the masseter and temporalis muscles. The patient may be asked to clench his jaw and the therapist palpates for the intensity of contraction of the masseter and temporalis muscles and compares with the opposite side. The patient is either unable or difficult to raise, depress, protrude, retract and deviate the mandible. The jaw is deflected to the affected side and the patient is unable to push it to the opposite side.

The jaw jerk, and corneal reflex are also tested.

- *Facial nerve:* The facial nerve is also a mixed nerve and therefore needs to be examined for its sensory and motor function. The facial nerve supplies all those muscles concerned with the facial expressions hence one should check the power of the frontalis, corrugator supercili, orbicularis oculi, nasalis, buccinator, rhizorios and orbicularis oris. The tone of the muscles for facial expression is observed and signs of atrophy as well as fasciculations are looked for. The reflexes tested are the corneal reflex, the orbicularis oculi reflex or glabellar reflex. Sensory examination of the facial nerve involves evaluation the taste sensation in the anterior two-third of the tongue. The four common flavors tested are sweet, salty, sour and bitter. The testing substance should be placed on the anterior two-third of the tongue and measures should be taken to prevent the solution from flowing on to the posterior aspect of the tongue or the opposite side. Thus the tongue should be held protruded and the patient should not speak.

- *The vestibulocochlear nerve:* This nerve comprises of two nerve in a single trunk. The cochlear nerve for hearing and the vestibular nerve for equilibrium, coordination and orientation in space. Before testing for hearing the external auditory canal should be examined with the otoscope to eliminate the presence of wax, pus, blood, foreign bodies, etc. Two tests are commonly performed, the Rinne test and Weber test. The Rinne test is for comparing the air and bone conduction. The tuning fork is placed against the mastoid process till the sound is no longer heard. It is then placed in front of the external auditory meatus and the time for which it is heard is noted. In normal individual or in positive Rinne's test the tuning fork is heard longer by air than bone. But in conductive deafness or negative Rinne's the air conduction is diminished and the bone conduction is retained. In sensorineural deafness both the air and bone conduction is diminished.

In Weber test the tuning fork is held on the vertex of the skull or center of the forehead. In normal individual it is heard equally well on both the side or there is no lateralization. If one ear is occluded then patient hears more on that side because the block in the ear has made it a resonating chamber. Thus in conductive deafness the sound is usually lateralized to the involved side but in sensorineural deafness the fork is heard best in the unaffected side.

Involvement of the vestibular part of the nerve is manifested by presence of vertigo, nystagmus or loss of balance. The Nylen-Barany maneuver for positional nystagmus and vertigo consists of making the patient lie down supine with the head off the bed extended at about 45 degree and laterally flexed at the same angle to both the sides will produce nystagmus and vertigo. Other tests like the rotation test, caloric test and galvanic test may be performed to evaluate the vestibular function.

- *Glossopharyngeal and vagus:* The patient may be asked to say "Aah" and the elevation of the soft palate on either side is noticed. The gag reflex, swallowing ability of the patient, etc. indicates the function of these two cranial nerve. The glossopharyngeal has sensory supplies to the posterior 1/3rd of the tongue which should be examined.
- *Accessory:* The power of the trapezius muscles on either side gives an idea about the function of the accessory nerve.
- *Hypoglossal nerve:* It supplies the tongue muscle. Hence, motor fibers can be checked by observing the movements of the tongue. It should be noted that during an act of tongue protrusion, the tongue muscles push the tongue out hence in case of weakness on one side the tongue will get deviated to the side of weakness.

Sensory Examination

Sensory examination are classified into three category for evaluation purpose as superficial, deep and cortical sensations.

- **Superficial sensation:** Superficial sensation comprises of the fine touch, crude touch, pinprick and thermal. They are checked along the dermatomal distribution over the body. Fine touch is checked with a wisp of cotton or edge of the cloth or feather. Crude touch is checked by the tip of the finger or any other blunt object. Pinprick is checked by a needle or any sharp object so that a minimal pressure evokes a distinct response of superficial pain. Thermal sensation may be checked by test tubes containing of warm and cold water or better with cold or warm metal tubes as glass in a poor conductor of temperature.

While assessing proper technique of implementation should be adopted to prevent any chances of manipulation by the patient and to obtain a clear-cut idea about the patient's level of sensory perception. Questions such as "Are you feeling anything" or "Do you feel now" should be totally avoided to prevent guesswork by the patient.

Technique

The therapist should instruct the patient to close the eyes and report the sensation as YES the moment he feel the sensation without waiting for the therapist to ask him. Stimulation with the appropriate object should be given alternately on both the side of the body at the same point for comparison. Once the therapist is convinced that the patient is appreciating the sensation without any signs of doubt then he should ask the patient to compare the sensation with the normal side. In case there is difference in the level of perception then the percentage of difference also needs to be specified as to 25 percent less or so. All the superficial sensations need to be checked.

- **Deep sensation:** Deep sensation comprises of the vibration sensation and the proprioceptive sensation. Deep pressure sensation can also be checked. Pallesthesia or sense of vibration is the ability to perceive the presence of vibration when an oscillating tuning fork is placed over certain bony prominence.

  Technique: A tuning fork of 128 Hz or 256 Hz is placed in vibration and held on the great toe or over the lateral or medial malleolus until the patient no longer feels it vibrate in these places. The patient should be able to perceive the fork with maximum vibration and should feel when it has almost stopped vibrating. The finding of normal vibratory threshold in the distal lower extremities can usually obviate the need for detailed testing either proximally or in the upper limb. Loss of vibratory sensation is termed as pallanesthesia.

  Joint position is tested in the distal most joint in the lower limb and the upper limb. Thus it is commonly tested in the IP joint of the big toe and the thumb. While checking the joint position sensation the therapist should hold the sides of the digit and not the pulp as it can help the patient in making use of the pressure or tactile sensation to guess the direction of movement.

Technique: The therapist shows the movements to the patient first and then asks him to close the eyes. The therapist holds the digit to be tested and moves it in different direction and asks the patient to identify the position with the eyes closed. In case the patient has a speech disturbance then he may be asked to position or move the digit of the adjoining limb in the similar fashion as that of the digit that is tested. In quadriplegics with speech involvement like in case of brainstem stroke, the eyeball movements can be used to indicate the patient level of perception for joint position.

Deep pressure although closely related to tactile sense involves perception of pressure from the subcutaneous structures rather than light touch from skin. Pressure sensation can be tested by firm pressure over the skin with a finger or blunt object with the eyes closed.

- **Cortical sensation:** Cortical sensation are developmental sensation which has occurred due to the learning and integration function of the brain. They are controlled by the sensory cortex and do not have a separate peripheral representation like the receptors or the nerve ending. They are a learned form of tactile sensation hence mediated by the same receptors and nerve fibers.

  Cortical sensation comprises of tactile localization, tactile discrimination and stereognosis (tactile agnosia), barognosia graphethesia.

  From practical point of view testing the tactile localization and stereognosis is sufficient for assessing one's cortical sensation abilities. Although tactile discrimination is ideally tested with the help of a pointed divider it gives rise to practical errors giving a false information about the patient's capabilities.

  Tactile localization is the ability of the patient to exactly point the area that is either pricked or touched by the therapist.

  Technique: The patient is asked to close the eyes, the therapist touches any one point on the part to be examined and ask the patient to point out the exact location, mere telling the part will no do, the patient should be insisted on localizing the exact site. Some patient may have the gross sensation and will be successful in coming close to the area of contact but will fail to exactly localize. Thus, the involvement of tactile localization may range from severe to mild involvement. Severe involvement is when the patient feels the touch sensation but are just not able to say whether in foot, arm, thigh, etc. Patient with mild involvement will be successful in telling the area like foot, arm, etc. but won't be able to point the exact site.

Stereognosis is the ability of a person to recognize familiar object with the help of tactile sensation.

Technique: The patient is asked to close the eyes and any familiar object is given in the hand of the patient without giving any form of auditory clue (sounds of object like key can give information to the patient). The patient is instructed to explore the object using the tactile sensation and come out with the correct guess. The person should be given a very familiar object and not the one which he must have not seen or used in his life.

Although, usually the assessment of the sensory system is done dermatome wise, but the final interpretation of the sensory deficit should be made taking into consideration four possibilities which are:

- Sensory deficit due to peripheral nerve injuries which is along the cutaneous distribution.
- Sensory deficit due to lesion in the spinal cord that is as per the affected spinal segment hence dermatomically.
- Sensory deficit due to involvement of the ascending tracts in the subcortical part of the brain like the brainstem or thalamus.
- Sensory deficit due to involvement of the sensory cortex of the brain which is as per the sensory homunculus.

Reflex Testing

The superficial and deep reflex should be tested. The common superficial reflex tested are plantar response, abdominal reflex, cremastic, and corneal reflex. The deep reflexes tested are deep tendon jerks like biceps, brachioradialis, triceps, knee jerks and ankle jerks.

Motor Examination

- *Tone:* Tone or tonus has been defined as the tension within the muscles when they are relaxed or as their resistance to passive movement when voluntary control is absent. The patient should be assessed to find out whether the tone in the muscles is normal or hypertonic or hypotonic. Hypertonic cases should also be differentiated for spasticity and rigidity.

In testing tone, the examiner should attempt to secure the complete cooperation of the patient. The patient should be comfortable and relaxed.

The most important criterion in the examination of tone is the resistance of muscles to passive manipulation when they are relaxed and when voluntary control is absent. In testing tone one examines passive and not active movement and notes the degree of tension or resistance offered by the muscles to passive stretching as well as the extensibility and range. There are other tests available which can be used to find the presence of hypertonicity in the patient like Babinski tonus test, Head dropping test, Pendulousness of the leg, Shoulder shaking test, Arm dropping test, etc. However the details of these tests are beyond the scope of this textbook as it is not essential for undergraduate studies.

- *Tightness:* The therapist should check for tightness of muscles of the lower extremities and upper extremities. Usually biarticular muscles are very prone to develop tightness. Muscles like Hamstring, Rectus femoris, Tendoachilles, Lateral flexor of the trunk, Adductor, Biceps, Long flexors of the hand should be assessed for tightness. During examination one should be skillful in demarcating tightness from spasticity. It is true that spastic muscles over a period of time can become tight, but both these are two different terms having a different meaning and should not be used a synonyms. Whether spasticity is an abnormal neurological condition, the term tightness represents a purely mechanical process that may be seen in normal also.

  While assessing for tightness the therapist should also find those muscles, which has gone into a contracture giving rise to deformity. This discrimination is necessary to be found, as there is difference in the type of physiotherapy approach for these two conditions while planning out the treatment protocol for the patient.

- *ROM:* The passive ROM for all the joints should be checked to rule out any mechanical or biomechanical constraint which interferes in the patient's level of functional independence.

- *MMT/voluntary control testing:* Manual muscle testing and voluntary control testing are two distinct examination procedures which should be done in all the neurological patients provided the patients cooperation can be obtained. As these are active procedures it cannot be done in unconscious patient, infants and mentally challenged individual. These procedures are two different methods having varied significance and one should know when to opt for either of them. Manual muscle testing is done to find the strength of the muscles in conditions with lower motor neuron like neuropathy, myopathy, anterior horn cell lesions, radiculopathy, etc. Isometric manual muscle testing should also be done in conditions where movements becomes difficult of perform and weakness is suspected like parkinsonism, ataxia, etc. Although these conditions have no direct influence on the muscle power but they cause generalize weakness called as asthenia due to deconditioning effect on the muscles.

MMT and voluntary control testing are a very detail practical procedure done for all muscles and movements respectively therefore cannot be described within the confinement of this chapter. The various grades used in these examination procedures are as follows:

MMT Grades
0 — No contraction.
1 — Flicker of contraction.
2 — Full range of motion in gravity eliminated plane.
3 — Full range of motion against gravity.
4 — Full range of motion against gravity and against half of maximal resistance.
5 — Full range of motion against gravity and against maximal resistance.

Grades of Voluntary Control Testing
0 — No contraction.
1 — Initiation of contraction or flicker of contraction.
2 — Half range of motion in pattern.
3 — Full range of motion in pattern.
4 — Initial half range in isolation and later half in pattern.
5 — Full range of motion in isolation but goes in pattern on giving resistance.
6 — Full range of motion in isolation and can take resistance like normals.

Unlike manual muscle testing where the therapist needs to stabilize the bone just proximal to the joint, in voluntary control the therapist gives an appropriate starting position, instructs the patient specifically and just observes the movement done. The starting position for testing voluntary control is usually the anti-synergistic position. For instance while testing for control of shoulder flexion, the therapist keeps the extremity in internal rotation, extension, elbow extension and forearm pronation, he then asks the patient to perform isolated shoulder flexion maintaining the antisynergistic attitude of the extremity. The grading is done after observing the manner by which the patient completes the task. Similarly for checking knee flexion, the patient is asked to lie in sidelying position, the hip is kept in extension and slight adduction. The patient is then asked to perform isolated flexion at the knee without performing any movement at the hip. This way all the joints are tested for all the movements.

Coordination Assessment

The various equilibrium and non-equilibrium test for incoordination are given in Chapter 3 Incoordination.

Perceptual Testing

The patient should be examined for visuospatial perception (which is relationship of various object with each other), identification of his body parts, discrimination of his body part from others, identifying an object from its background especially if they have the same color (figure ground discrimination), geographical orientation (identification of familiar places), and discrimination between right and left side. These are some of the basic perceptual functions that needs to be assessed by the therapist.

Balance Testing

Each moment of our life, we adopt so many different position and each position needs a different combination of neuromuscular work for which proper postural mechanism is necessary. Postural mechanism and balance are inseparable from each other. Without balance it is impossible for us to perform various task be it static or dynamic. Balance forms the necessary background or foundation with the help of which we perform various task. Hence the assessment of balance is very essential for neurologically disabled patient.

Some of the common tests that are used consists of :
- Romberg test
- Sharpened Romberg test (In tandem stance attitude)
- Postural sway test
- Nudge or perturbation test
- Functional reach test
- Multidirectional reach test
- Berg balance test
- Get up and go test.

There are still some other test which may be used but are beyond the scope of this textbook.

Romberg Test

Romberg test consists of making the patient stand with feet parallel to each other with a normal width between the feet and then close the eyes for 20 to 30 seconds. The therapist observes for the sway. Mild sway is present even in normal individual for first few seconds immediately as the visual feed back is cut off but a normal person stabilizes immediately following mild initial sway. But a patient with postural column disease who primarily depends upon the visual sensation will sway maximally and may even fall. If the patient sways even with eyes open then it indicates a gross balance deficit and could be due to lesion to the cerebellum.

Sharpened Romberg

Sharpened Romberg consists of the patient to stand with the feet in a tandem stance attitude (heel of front foot in contact with the toe of the back foot), arm folded across the chest and stand for about one minute.

One Leg Stance

One leg stance consists of testing both the legs alternately in a unilateral stance attitude to find out the difference in the level of stability on weight bearing individually on both the legs. The patient may be given 5 trials with 30 seconds in each trial to stand without a fall. However even normal elderly person may find it difficult to stand on one leg stance continuously for 30 seconds.

In both Romberg test and one-legged stance test if the patient uses visual input to stabilize himself then he will immediately loose the balance on closing the eyes.

Timed Stance

Timed stance test consists of making the patient stand in various foot position like apart, together, tandem and single leg with eyes open and then with eyes closed thus giving rise to 8 different combinations. Maintenance of balance should be for a maximum of 30 seconds. Thus the maximum score a person can get is 240 second.

Postural Sway Test

Postural sway test consists of the use of computerized force plate on which the person is asked to stand in normal manner for about 20 to 30 seconds. Sway with both eyes open and with eyes closed is often measured. The computer provides with the graphical and numerical quantification.

Nudge Test

Nudge test is the most commonly used method for testing balance as it is very simple and can be quickly done. However it is very subjective and cannot quantify the various parameters hence cannot be used for documentation. It involves giving perturbation to the patient forward-backward as well as sideways and observing the patient's response to the pushes or perturbation. Perturbation should be given both while the patient is aware that you are going to push him and also when he is not expecting a push because this way we can check the patient's anticipatory response as well as his ability of automatic adaptations.

Functional Reach Test

In functional reach test, the client is asked to reach forward as far as possible from a comfortable standing posture. The excursion of the arm from the start to finish is measured via a yardstick affixed to the wall at the shoulder height. One of the limitation of the functional reach test is that it measures the sway in only one direction. Also since the patient takes support of the yard stick the biomechanical alignment of the body parts changes consequently there is a different balance reaction as compared to normal standing without support. Multidirectional reach test which is a modified type of functional reach test measures the sway in anteroposterior, medial and lateral direction provides more comprehensive data of voluntary balancing ability but the reliability is not known as it is a new test.

Berg Balance Test

Berg balance test consist of 14 different functional tasks which the patient needs to perform the therapist grades the performance of each task with the scores ranging from 0 to 4 . "0" is for unable to perform and "4" is for ability to perform without difficulty. The tasks consists of:

- Sitting to standing
- Standing unsupported for 2 minutes without holding on to an external support.
- Sitting unsupported with feet on floor for 2 minutes
- Standing to sitting
- Transfers
- Standing unsupported with eyes closed for 10 seconds.
- Standing unsupported with feet together
- Reaching forward with outstretched arm
- Pick up object from the floor
- Turning to look behind over the left and right shoulder
- Turn 360 degrees
- Count number of times the step stool is touched with the foot
- Standing unsupported one foot in front
- Standing on one leg.

The limitation of this test is that it test various tasks which requires the patient anticipatory control but does not test any activity which needs the automatic or reactive postural control (automatic adaptation).

Get up and Go test

The Get up and Go test was developed as a quick screening tool for detecting balance problems affecting daily mobility skills in elderly patients. In this test the patient is asked to stand up from a chair, walk 3 meters, turn around and return. Performance is scored according to the following scale: 1 is normal, 2 is very slightly abnormal, 3 is mildly abnormal, 4 is moderately abnormal and 5 is severely abnormal.

However most of the tests have limitations as they don't consider all the basic activity performed and the various environment in which they are performed normally. For instance the demand for balance during walking on even, uneven, crowded environment is totally different and such facts should not be ignored while assessing a patient's balance.

Gait Examination

To begin with one should observe whether the patient is walking independently or with assistance. Description of the assistance is better as the patient may use an aid either for only balance or may be using for weight bearing. The gait of the neurological disabled person should be checked for various parameters like step length, step width, stride length, stance time on each leg, and cadence. The therapist should check whether the patient has all the components of the normal gait in the stance and swing phase. Lastly the therapist should assess the kinematics and kinetics at various joints in the lower limb. The attitude of various body parts also needs to be described as the alignment of the whole body directly influences ones gait.

Examination of Autonomous Nervous System

The main autonomous function which is usually assessed is sweat function. Sweat function can be assessed by ninhydrin test or galvanic skin resistance test. Ninhydrin is a powder which is sprayed on the body part that needs to be examined. When it comes in contact with sweat it changes its color thus the part which has impaired sweating will not show any change in the color of ninhydrin powder sprayed over it. Galvanic skin resistance test will indicate lack of sweat by showing an increase in the skin impedance when current is passed through it.

Examination of autonomous nervous system is essential in spinal cord disorders, neuropathy and peripheral nerve injuries.

Functional Assessment

The activities of daily living such as feeding, dressing, hygiene, mobility and transfer needs to be assessed in detail. Infact the patient is more interested in seeing himself perform as much activities of daily living possible independently. Various way of grading has been followed like Barthel index, Katz index of ADL, the functional independence measure (FIM) and the outcome and assessment information set (OASIS). It is up to the therapist interest to follow anyone of this scale to rate the patient's level of independence because then comparison becomes easier in the later stage to determine the extent of prognosis the patient has achieved with a specific treatment. The author follows the last of these that is OASIS which grades grooming, dressing, bathing, toileting, transferring, ambulation, feeding, preparing light meals, transportation, laundry, housekeeping, and shopping into various grades depending upon whether the patient is independent or he needs assistance.

SELF-ASSESSING QUESTIONS

- Tests for various cranial nerves.
- Grades of MMT.
- Grades of voluntary control.
- Tests for assessing balance.
- Coordination tests.

2

Stroke

Stroke is defined as a sudden neurological deficit caused by focal vascular lesion in the brain.

The vascular lesion can be either a hemorrhagic or ischemic involving the blood vessels supplying various parts of the brain. The extent of neurological involvement may range from mild motor deficit to gross involvement of various function namely sensorimotor, perceptual, emotional, behavioral, memory, intelligence, speech and language function.

ETIOLOGY

Different mechanisms have been found to cause vascular insufficiency to the brain resulting in stroke. However, the most common causes are:

1. *Thrombus:* This is mainly due to the presence of atherosclerotic plaque in the cerebral arteries as a result of severe platelet adhesion, fibrinous coagulation and decreased fibrinolysis activity.

2. *Emboli:* These are free flowing bodies in the cerebral blood stream in the form of dislodged thrombus, fats, air, tissue particle, etc. which gets trapped at any point along their course, frequently at the bifurcation of the arteries, and cause occlusion to the cerebral circulation.

3. *Hemorrhage:* It occurs due to rupture of the blood vessels in the brain. Following hemorrhage tissue death occurs due to both ischemia and mechanical injury to the brain substance as a result of compression by the clot. Hemorrhage usually occurs either due to hypertension, arteriovenous malformation or even due to trauma.

There are some risk factors that can predispose to stroke. The common ones are diabetes, high blood pressure, and cardiac disorders. The chances of these three occurring in combination increases with age. Patients with increased hematocrit count are at a higher risk of getting stroke. Cardiac disorders like valvular heart diseases, endocarditis, atrial fibrillation, or postcardiac surgery patients are at a higher risk of contacting stroke. Other secondary risk factors that can increase the chances of stroke attack are cigarette smoking, obesity, sedentary lifestyle, increased consumption of high fat diet, psychological stress, and excessive alcohol intake.

PATHOPHYSIOLOGY OF CEREBRAL ISCHEMIA AND CONSEQUENT INFARCTION

The two pathophysiological changes leading to cerebral infarction are loss in the supply of oxygen and glucose due to vascular occlusion, and various changes in cellular metabolism consequent as a result of collapse of energy producing processes with disintegration of cell membranes.

Complete occlusion to brain substance causes severe damage to it with a zone of infarction, which is however found to be smaller than the actual area supplied by the involved artery. *The margin of this infarcted zone consists of cells that are alive but metabolically less active. These surrounding areas are termed as* **ischemic prenumbra**. These areas are nourished by meningeal collateral.

The necrotic tissue swells rapidly mainly due to excessive inter-cellular and intracellular water content. Also, lack of O_2 is another factor that can contribute to swelling.

This vascular lesion to the brain causes release of neuro-transmitters like glutamate and aspartate by the ischemic cells, which excites neurons and produces an intracellular influx of Na and Ca leading to irreversible cell damage. Thus recent research attempts at blocking this action of glutamatic and aspartate on nearby cells, which will reduce the secondary involvement of surrounding viable cells.

Cerebral edema begins within few minutes and reaches a maximum by about 4 days, however it mostly disappears by 3 weeks. This edema can increase the intracranial pressure and can even cause contralateral and caudal shift of brain structure (Fig. 2.1).

Neurovascular Syndromes

Internal carotid artery occlusion in its proximal segment immediately after its generation from the common carotid artery is often silent.

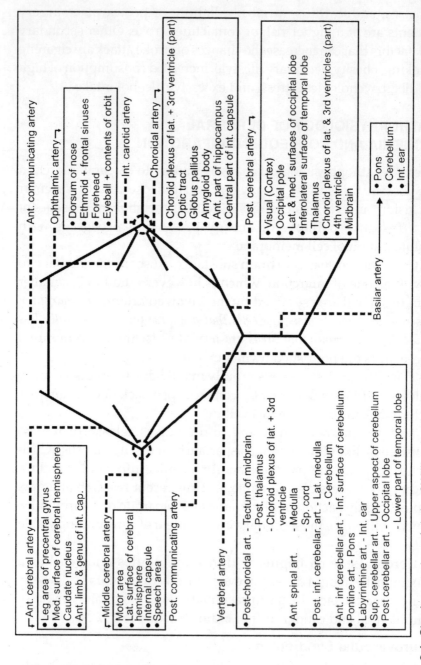

Fig. 2.1: Circulus arteriosus/ circle of Willis, showing distribution of various arteries and its blood supply to various areas in the brain

Middle Cerebral Artery

Structures involved	Neurological deficit
Motor area of face, arm, and fibers descending from leg area to enter the coronal radiata	Paralysis of contralateral face, arm and leg
Somatosensory area of face, arm and face leg	Sensory impairment over contralateral and leg
Motor (Broca's) area on dominant hemisphere	Motor speech disorder
Central language area and parieto-occipital cortex of the dominant hemisphere	Central aphasia, word deafness, anomia, jargon speech, alexia, agraphia, acalculia, and finger agnosia
Non-dominant parietal lobe	Perceptual disorder like unilateral neglect, anosognosial unwareness of hemiplegic side, apraxia, and spatial disorganization
	Homonymous hemianopia and loss of conjugate gaze to the opposite side
Parietal lobe	Ataxia of contralateral limbs
Bilateral frontal lobe	Brun's ataxia or apraxia of gait
Supramarginal gyrus or inferior parietal lobe	Loss or impairment of optokinetic nystagmus
Posterior limb of internal capsule and adjacent corona radiata	Pure motor hemiplegia without sensory and visual involvement

Infarction secondary to proximal MCA occlusion often produces significant cerebral edema with increased intracranial pressures and may lead to brain herniation, coma or death.

Anterior Cerebral Artery

Structure involved	Neurological deficit
Motor leg area	Paralysis of opposite foot and leg
Involvement of arm area	Involvement of opposite arm although this is rare
Sensory area of foot and arm	Cortical sensory loss over foot and leg

Contd...

Contd...

Structure involved	Neurological deficit
Bilateral involvement of posteromedial part of superior frontal gyrus	Urinary incontinence
Medial surface of posterior frontal lobe	Contralateral grasp reflex, sucking reflex and gegenhalten (paratonic rigidity), frontal tremor
Severe frontal lobe infarction	Memory loss and behavioral impairments
Supplementary motor area of dominant hemisphere	Aphasia
Corpus callosum	Apraxia and agraphia
Bilateral motor area of leg	Cerebral hemiplegia

Homonymous hemianopia never occurs in ACA stroke.

Posterior Cerebral Artery

Structure involved	Neurological deficit
Thalamus	Hemianesthesia (contralateral sensory loss) or thalamic sensory syndromes (unpleasant hemibody sensation with spontaneous pain)
Occipital cortex	Homonymous hemianopia, visual agnosia, prosopagnosia
Bilateral occipital cortex involvement	Cortical blindness
Temporal lobe ischemia	Amnesic syndrome with memory defect
Midbrain	Skew deviation, athetoid posturing, postural tremor, hemiballismus)
Cerebral peduncle	Contralateral hemiplegia
Motor tract between red and vestibular nuclei	Decerebrate attacks

Vertebrobasilar Artery

The basilary artery supplies the pons, inner ear and cerebellum. Complete occlusion is often fatal. Progressive lesion often starts with occipital headache, and then causes diplopia, hemiplegia, quadriplegia and finally coma.

Locked in syndrome is seen in lesion involving the ventral pontine nuclei with a complete basilar syndrome without affection of the reticular system and is described as anarthria, quadriplegia, but preserved consciousness. Alertness and gaze are intact, infact the only communication that can be established is through vertical eye movements. Prognosis of this condition is very poor and the residual disability in surviving population is severe.

Vertebrobasilar artery system occlusion can produce either ipsilateral or contralateral symptoms depending upon whether the tracts involved indirectly have already crossed or uncrossed. Cranial nerve abnormalities along with cerebellar symptoms can occur. Symptoms such as visual loss, homonymous hemianopia, diplopia, facial numbness, or weakness, tinnitus, dysarthria, or dysphagia may be seen.

Hemiparesis of one or more limbs can occur with involvement of corticospinal tract.

Paresthesia of the face or limbs can occur with involvement of the leminiscal system. Pain and temperature sensation on the opposite side will be involved in the ischemia of the spinothalamic tract involvement.

Reticular spinal tract involvement causes alteration in the level of consciousness. Horner's syndrome due to sympathetic tract involvement is rare. *Sudden loss of tone in the lower limbs as a result of involvement of the medullary pyramids is termed as Drop attack* can also result in vertebrobasilar artery syndrome.

TIA (transient ischemic attack) due to affection of vertebrobasilar artery is very common than carotid artery.

CLINICAL MANIFESTATION

Sensory

The sensory involvement in a stroke patient depends upon the site and the extent of the lesion. Touch, pain, temperature, proprioceptive sensation may be involved to a variable degree. The affection of these sensation is more in case of the lesion involving the thalamus which can even cause *contralateral hemianesthesia*. Involvement of the somatosensory area of the cortex causes loss of cortical sensation namely *tactile localization, tactile discrimination, stereognosis,* and *tactile extinction* (which is inability to appreciate the stimulus on the affected side when it is applied simultaneously with the stimulus on the unaffected side, although the patient does perceives the sensation when the stimulus is applied alternately).

A common visual disturbances seen is *homonymous hemianopia* in which there is loss of vision in the nasal half of opposite eye and the temporal half of the eye on the hemiplegic side. This usually occurs due to lesion of the optic radiation in the internal capsule or primary visual cortex.

Crossed anesthesia can be seen if the lesion involves the upper part of the pons in which there is anesthesia on the same side of the face and on the opposite side of the trunk and limbs.

Lack of *Conjugate gaze* may be noted.

Motor

Immediately after the onset of stroke, there is a stage of cerebral shock with flaccidity and areflexia. Gradually, this is replaced by development of spasticity, hyperreflexia, and abnormal mass movement pattern, which is termed as synergy.

The duration of flaccidity may vary from days to weeks to infinite. In some rare cases (conditions in which there is pure pyramidal tract lesion) signs of mild spasticity may be seen in certain groups of muscles like elbow flexors, wrist flexors, quadriceps and calf, but total predominating spasticity never sets in.

However majority of the cases go through a common sequence of prognosis, which according to Brunstorm comprised of five stages (Table 2.1). This was further simplified by Bobath into only three stages (Table 2.2). Thus it is clear that 95 percent of hemiplegics show spontaneous recovery although the degree of the recovery may vary depending upon various factors, and the progress may become stagnant at any point of time.

This development of hypertonicity has been termed as a positive reaction by Jacksonian as it enables the patient to gain some level of dependency. The other response is a negative response, which occurs due to disruption of the higher facilitatory influence on the spinal

Table 2.1: Stages according to Brunstorm

Stage 1	Flaccid and no movements
Stage 2	Spasticity begins and basic limb synergies may be seen as associated reaction
Stage 3	Limb synergies are produced voluntarily
Stage 4	Some movement combination not belonging to synergy may appear, spasticity starts declining
Stage 5	More difficult movement combinations are learned if improvement
Stage 6	Spasticity disappears, isolated movement possible and coordination also can become normal

Table 2.2: Bobath's stage

1. Flaccid
2. Spastic
3. Stage of spontaneous recovery

nerves. The negative response gives rise to weakness or paresis, which is however masked by the predominant spasticity in the patient.

Spasticity

Severe degree of spasticity will make movements impossible; moderate spasticity will allow for some slow movements but they will be performed with too much effort and abnormal coordination; mild spasticity will allow for gross movements with normal coordination but fine movements of the limbs especially involving the distal portion will be difficult or impossible.

In hemiparesis there are some muscles which are always involved and which consequently give rise to a peculiar abnormal mass movement pattern and attitude that is characteristic of many hemiparesis patient. The spasticity invariably affects the antigravity muscle for reasons not clearly understood. It is however presumed that this antigravity muscle are relatively more stretched than progravity muscles in neutral position hence stimulating the stretch reflex giving rise to spasticity.

The distribution of spasticity in the upper and lower extremities is as follows (Table 2.3):

Table 2.3: Distribution of spasticity in upper and lower extremities

Upper extremities	Lower extremities
1. Shoulder girdle: depressor and retractor	1. Pelvic girdle: retractor
2. Shoulder: internal rotators and adductors	2. Hip: extensor, adductor, and internal rotators
3. Elbow: Flexors	3. Knee: Extensors
4. Wrist and finger: Flexor	4. Ankle and toes: Plantar flexors and supinators
5. Forearm: pronators	

Spasticity also involves the muscles of the trunk and neck on the opposite side causing lateral bending of patient towards the spastic side

Synergy

Synergy patterns are abnormal, stereotyped, primitive, mass movement pattern associated with spasticity and which can be triggered either reflexly or voluntarily.

Synergy can be either flexor or extensor. They involve the action of certain muscles in combination that gives rise to an abnormal movement pattern not useful for functional activities. This abnormal synergies are presented in Table 2.4.

Table 2.4: Abnormal synergies in upper and lower limbs

	Upper limbs	Lower limbs
Flexion synergy	Shoulder girdle retraction and elevation, shoulder abduction external rotation, supination flexion of elbow, wrist and finger flexion	Hip flexion abduction and lateral rotation, knee flexion, dorsiflexion and inversion
Extension synergy	Shoulder girdle protraction and depression, shoulder adduction, internal rotation, elbow extension, pronation wrist and finger flexion	Hip extension, adduction, internal rotation, knee extension, ankle plantar flexion, inversion and toe plantar flexion

Thus it can observed that the following muscles does not take part in either of the synergies.
a. Latissimus dorsi
b. Teres major
c. Serratus anterior
d. Wrist and finger extensors
e. Ankle evertors

It is highly essential to understand that synergies are different from the abnormal attitude seen in a hemiparesis patient. The abnormal hemiplegic attitude is due to the combination of strongest component of the flexor and extensor synergy in both upper and lower limbs. The strongest components for the upper limb in the flexor synergy are shoulder girdle retraction, elbow flexion, wrist and finger flexion. The strongest components of the extensor synergy for the upper limb are shoulder girdle depression, shoulder adduction, internal rotation, and pronation.

The strongest components of the flexor synergy for the lower limb are lateral rotation, and inversion. The strongest components of the extensor synergy for the lower limbs are pelvic retraction, hip adduction, hip extension, knee extension and plantar flexion.

Hence, a hemiplegic patient has an attitude of shoulder retraction and depression, shoulder adduction and internal rotation, elbow flexion, pronation and wrist and finger flexion. The lower limb adopts an attitude of pelvic retraction, hip extension, adduction and external rotation, knee extension, and ankle plantar flexion and inversion. This is shown in the Figure 2.2 (Plate 1).

Reflexes

In the stage of flaccidity all the reflexes are suppressed or absent. As the patient enters into the stage of spasticity, the reflexes reoccur. The deep tendon reflexes become hyperactive, infact, in case of increased spasticity there may be presence of clonus especially of the tendo Achilles and wrist flexors. Superficial reflexes are lost but plantar responses show Babinski sign positive.

Release of primitive reflexes: Due to the lesion in the brain the other primitive reflexes that are produced by the lower level of CNS are released from the inhibitory influences of the higher centers. The common primitive reflexes that are seen in a hemiplegics are ATNR (Asymmetrical tonic neck reflexes)—Rotation of the head to one side causes extension and adduction on the same side and flexion and abduction on the opposite side.

   i. *Symmetrical tonic neck reflex (STNR)* Flexion of the head causes flexion of the upper extremities and extension of the lower extremities. Extension of the head causes extension of the upper extremities and flexion of the lower extremities.

ii. *Symmetrical tonic labyrinthine Reflex (STLR)* Supine position causes a increase in extensor tone and prone position increase the tone in the flexor muscles.

iii. *Tonic lumbar reflex (TLR)* Rotation of the trunk to the hemiplegic side over the pelvis causes flexion of the hemiplegic upper limb and extension of the hemiplegic lower limbs. Rotation to the opposite side causes the opposite effect.

iv. *Flexor withdrawal* Sensory stimulation to the sole of the foot causes a sudden hip-knee flexion. Infact in some patient this may be so dominating that it may interfere in the assessment of plantar response.

v. *Positive supporting reaction* Pressure at the bottom of the foot causes co-contraction of the lower limb muscles making the limb like a rigid pillar.

Associated Reaction

Associated reactions are tonic postural reaction in muscles. They are abnormal reaction, which usually manifest itself as an attenuation of the hemiplegic's attitude in response to movement either on the same side of the body or occurring in any other parts. These abnormal positioning of the limb becomes very obvious during ambulation. These abnormal associated reactions should be differentiated from the normal associated movements (also called synkinetic movements), e.g. swinging of the arm while walking.

Impairment of Higher Level Reactions

Reflexes that are controlled by higher level of the brain like, righting reactions, equilibrium reactions, automatic adaptations of the muscles to the change of postures are all impaired.

Righting reactions: These are automatic responses which maintain the normal position of the head, trunk and limbs with respect to their alignment to each other. They help in carrying out various functions like rolling, getting up, sitting and standing.

Equilibrium reactions: These are normal responses, which help us in maintaining the balance during all our activities especially when we are in a danger of falling.

Automatic adaptation in postural tone: The automatic adjustment that takes place in order to allow for normal movement or maintenance of posture is termed as automatic postural tone. Examples: The contraction of erector spinae while bending forward and thus preventing a fall. Eccentric contraction of the quadriceps muscle while squatting is another example of automatic adjustment of the muscles. Similarly synergistic fixation of the proximal parts to allow movement to take place distally is also an example of postural adaptation of muscles.

Also in hemiplegics there may be impairment of *protective reactions* like extension of the upper limbs to avoid injuries during a fall.

Speech and Language Disorders

This occurs due to lesion involving the dominant parietal lobe. Three types of speech disorders have been seen following a stroke.

Broca's/motor/expressive/non-fluent aphasia: In this type of aphasia the patient's ability to understand is intact, but his ability to respond is affected due to involvement of the Broca's area. He has difficulty in articulating his speech.

Wernicke's/sensory/receptive/fluent aphasia: The patient's ability to speak is intact, infact his speech is very fluent, but he doesn't understand or comprehend. His speech is totally irrelevant.

Global/conductive or total aphasia: In this type there is loss of understanding as well as production of speech. This occurs due to lesion of both the Broca's and Wernicke's area or may be due to the involvement of the conduction zone between these two.

Apraxia and Agnosia

Apraxia is inability to carry out learned purposeful movement despite the presence of a good motor, sensory, or coordination function. It is caused due to lesion of the dominant parietal lobe. Bilateral apraxia commonly involves lips and tongue. When the patient is asked to purse the lips or protrude the tongue, he won't be able to do it. But the patient may be found doing the same while having food. Thus movements are performed spontaneously but not on command. There are three types of apraxia noted.

Ideomotor is the type in which patient understands the purpose of movement but is unable to carry out on command but does it automatically.

Ideational is characterized by extreme absent-mindedness. Patient fails to perform purposeful movement both spontaneously and on command.

Constructional apraxia is difficulty in spatial organization of movement or objects, e.g. inability to imitate simple arrangements of blocks or a simple drawing.

Agnosia is failure to recognize objects despite having an intact visual, auditory, and tactile sensation, due to the lack of association pathways to arrange sensory images, memory and disposition towards the action.

Visual agnosia is inability to recognize common objects which is seen clearly by the patient due to lesion in the dominant parieto-occipital regions.

Auditory agnosia is inability to recognize familiar sounds or music due to lesion of dominant temporal lobe although the patient has an intact hearing.

Tactile agnosia is inability to recognize object by using hand although there is no sensory defect in the hand. This occurs due to lesion involving the dominant parietal lobe.

A special form of agnosia is Autotopagnosia in which patient fails to recognize different part of the body. Infact, he may deny that his body parts belong to him.

Anosognosia is unawareness of hemiplegic side. The autotopagnosia and anosognosia occurs due the lesion involving the dominant lobe thus affecting the opposite side of the body.

Lesion of the inferior region of the dominant parietal cortex causes confusion between right and left finger agnosia (unable to identify finger when touched), agraphia (difficulty in writing), and acalculia (inability to calculate). This is called as *Gerstmann's syndrome*.

Perception and Cognitive Dysfunction

Perception dysfunction occur due to lesion of the non-dominant parietal lobe.

The perceptual impairment could be in the form of visuospatial disorders, unilateral body neglect, somatognosia or visual perceptual impairment.

Visuospatial relation disorder: It is difficulty in determining the distance, size, position, and relationship of various parts to the whole. An individual reaching out for an object may over estimate or underestimate the distance, e.g: If the individual has to wash his hand, he may hold the hand next to the tap instead of keeping under it. Also as he is unable to judge the distance the individual have been found to constantly collide with the wall or doorway.

Unilateral body neglect or inattention: The individual does not use the involved limb, i.e. the non-dominant limb, to its available control and infact ignores it. An individual with unilateral body neglect will wash the unaffected side of the body properly but not the affected side. Similarly, other activities like combing, clothing, shaving, face wash, etc. are done in same fashion.

Visuospatial impairment: In this impairment the individual does not respond to or recognize any meaningful stimuli which is present in the side contralateral to the affected non-dominant hemisphere, e.g. for a right dominant individual, the left side of the space appears not to be seen. The patient may eat only that part of the food kept on the right side of the plate. Also, while reading the newspaper the patient will read only that matter which is present on the right side of the page.

Somatognosia: This is also called body scheme or body image dysfunction. The patient will be unable to differentiate between mirror image and self. The individual may attempt to comb his mirror image instead of himself. Also, the patient may not be able to differentiate between his own body parts and that of others, hence, he may try to wear a watch in someone else wrist.

Visual perceptual impairment: Distortion in the perception of vertical and horizontal plane, which leads to frequent falling. Also, the patient have topographical disorientation (difficulty in finding way from one place to another). He will also have difficulty in telling time, visualizing mental picture of familiar person and figure ground impairment (inability to differentiate an object from the back ground).

Cognitive and behavioral changes occurs in lesion involving. either of the cerebral hemisphere. *Patients with left hemisphere damage are usually very depressed, low profile, anxious and have a negative attitude towards life.* They are often cautious, insecure, slow in their movement and hesitant in their approach towards any activity. These patients need lot of encouragement and positive feedback from the therapist.

Patients with right hemisphere lesion are often euphoric, overconfident, impulsive and over estimate their capability. They often deny that they are disabled and hence the chance of causing injury is more in these individuals. They have to be trained to perform the movement with more caution and slow manner.

Cognitive dysfunction also manifests as difficulty in orientation, attention, conceptual abilities, memory and learning. Short-term memory is usually affected.

Dysphagia

The correlation of stroke with dysphagia remains unclear. However, it has been proved that dysphagia is quite frequently noted in patients with bilateral cerebral hemisphere or brainstem lesion. It is caused only when stroke involves larger cerebral vessels. Dysphagia frequently causes aspiration, which may need hospitalization or even death. The most common reason for aspiration is incomplete laryngeal elevation and closure. Altered sensation, palatal paralysis, defective lip closure and postural imbalance have all been contributing towards dysphagia.

Bladder and Bowel Impairment

In flaccid stage there is overflow incontinence hence continuous catheterization is advisable. Anterior communicating artery strokes involving paracentral lobule can cause loss of voluntary control of micturition. The patient will have sudden uncontrolled evacuation of urination irrespective of the time and place. Also there may be presence of constipation. However, no detail work has been carried out on this disability.

Sexual Dysfunction

Sexual activity is important for many couples throughout their lives. Many individuals are worried about their sexual life but are hesitant or shy to discuss or seek advice for the same.

Stroke may interfere with the sexual activity by affecting the individual desire, libido, erectile or lubrication, orgasm or ejaculation. The disability could be due to depressed state, sensorimotor dysfunction, etc.

Secondary Manifestation

Psychological Dysfunction

Psychological dysfunction are very common after an attack of stroke and are usually manifested as depression, social withdrawal, anxiety, sleep disorder (insomnia), secondary mania, emotional lability (pathological crying and laughing, emotional incontinence), behavior problem (aggressiveness, verbal abusing or yelling, resistive behavior or over dependency) and even personality changes like an introvert can become extrovert and may appear very happy and over talkative.

Musculoskeletal Complications

Musculoskeletal complications set in 95 percent of stroke patients if proper physiotherapy treatment is not given. It occurs mainly due to the combination of muscular imbalance and inactivity. Pain and stiffness are the common ones that affect various joints. However, certain joints are frequently involved like wrist flexors, elbow flexors, shoulder adductor, pronator, plantar flexor, knee extensor, and unilateral tightness of neck and trunk lateral flexors on the spastic side.

Decreased tone in the flaccid stage commonly causes subluxation of the glenohumoral joint on affected side if adequate care is not taken. This subluxation if allowed to persist may even give rise to periarthritis or frozen shoulder in subacute stages.

Pain at the shoulder can trigger the incidence of RSD (reflex sympathetic dystrophy or shoulder hand syndrome), which is abnormally increased sympathetic overflow. It occurs in three stages. Stage I manifested by burning pain and paresthesia, pitting edema (commonly on the dorsum of hand), decrease in wrist flexion range, cyanosis of hand due to vasoconstriction and increased sweating. Stage II in which there is increased pain, decrease in sweating, warm and more firmer hand, osteoporosis involving the bones of the limbs. Stage III gives rise to indurated edema, atrophy of the bones and the muscles. Pain is usually absent in this stage, the hand becomes cool and deformity occurs due to involvement of the soft tissue around the joints. Claw hand deformity is very commonly seen. Hence close observation by the therapist is essential to prevent the progression into the third stage.

Scalenus anticus syndrome occurs because the patient continuously assumes a posture of head flexion, shoulder internal rotation, scapula retraction. It is manifested as neck and shoulder discomfort with tingling numbness in the hand and fingers.

Deep Vein Thrombosis (DVT)

Deep veins thrombosis in stroke is not as common as in spinal cord injury. It occurs due to accumulation of the clot in the distal blood vessels. It is manifested as pain or tenderness in the calf muscle, swelling, and discoloration of the leg. It can occur in hemiplegia mainly if the patient remains in comatose state for a long time.

Cardiac and Respiratory Deconditioning

Although the cardiac and respiratory systems are not directly affected, decreased physical activity has been found out to be the main cause of deconditioning of these systems. The patient's endurance level is drastically reduced which may adversely affect the rehabilitation process.

Pain

Pain is very common only in stroke affecting the thalamus and is termed as thalamic syndrome, which is characterized by very intense burning pain on the opposite side of body. Pain can also occur as a result of various musculoskeletal complications as discussed above.

Gastrointestinal and Renal Systems

Although, these systems may not be directly involved, rarely, some patients with stroke do exhibit constipation and urinary tract infection or calculus. However the frequency of involvement is very low.

Comparison of Normal and Hemiplegic Gait

Walking is an independent, automatic, symmetrical and economical event. During a normal walking there is both vertical and horizontal

displacement of CG in the form of a sinusoidal wave that causes horizontal displacement of 1.7 inch and vertical displacement of 1.8 inch. The gait determinants are as follows:
- Knee flexion at heel strike on loading which lowers the CG
- Pelvic tilting
- Pelvic rotation which increases with increase in the heel strike
- Foot ankle mechanism
- Knee flexion on heel rise or heel off
- Lateral displacement of pelvis.

Under normal circumstances walking is an automatic process which requires contribution and integration of various mechanism, however after the brain damage like in cases of stroke all the automatic adaptation is lacking and the patient tries to compensate for it by putting more voluntary efforts. The phasic action of muscle groups seen normally is replaced by abnormal muscular combination characteristic of primitive reflexes. The flexion and extension synergy interferes with the walking and greatly influence the hemiplegic gait.

The abnormality of gait in hemiplegic patient can be compared with normal gait taking into consideration the contribution of the joints for various phases of the gait cycle.

Ankle Joint

Early stance (heel strike to foot flat): In normals when the heel strike the ground, the angle at the ankle is 90 degrees once the weight is transmitted to the fore foot, the sole is gradually lowered which is controlled by eccentric contraction of the dorsiflexors to prevent slapping of the foot.

In hemiplegics, the anticipation of the weight bearing excites the extensor synergy which induces plantar flexion instead of dorsiflexion because dorsiflexion is not a part of the extensor synergy. The hemiplegic limb comes down on the entire sole and if the plantar flexion is marked then on the toes. Thus the heel strike is completely missing in hemiplegics. If there is pronounced inversion there is more weight borne by the lateral aspect of the foot and when it is moderate it gets corrected on weight bearing.

Mid stance: In normal when the sole is firm on the ground the leg starts pivoting forwards above the ankle causing a relative dorsiflexion. This happens in response to the weight shift from hindfoot to the forefoot. The movement of relative dorsiflexion is controlled by eccentric work of the plantar flexors which gets gradually elongated.

In hemiplegics when the calf muscle is stretched by body weight it stimulates the stretch reflex causing increase spasticity of plantar flexors and it prevents any further stretch. Thus the forward shift of the body weight is prevented in hemiplegics.

Late stance (unloading to push off): In normals towards the end of the stance phase the heel raises from ground and the knee flexes. This is achieved by forceful concentric contraction of the plantar flexors for initiating a forward swing.

In hemiplegics, the knee does not flex due to lack of dorsiflexion at the ankle in the earlier phase and also due to the influence of quadriceps spasticity. Sometimes even if it does flex it flexes gradually. Moreover the combination of plantar flexion with knee flexion neither belongs to flexion or extension synergy hence is very difficult for a hemiplegic gait. Due to the lack of push off in hemiplegics the force required to initiate a swing is very less that causes slowness in walking.

Knee Joint

Early and midstance: In normals as the heel strikes the ground the knee is extended but as the body weight shifts on to the loading foot there is 15 degree flexion at the knee under the influence of body weight and it is controlled by eccentric contraction of the quadriceps to prevent buckling. Immediately afterwards due to concentric work of the quadriceps there is extension at the knee.

In hemiplegics patient in flaccid stage there can be bucking due to weight transmission. In stage of spasticity, the initial flexion does not take place and the knee continues to remain in hyperextension throughout. Some patient do have a tendency to buckle initially but immediately rectify by going into hyperextension.

Late stance: In normals the knee flexes with plantar flexion to a give momentum to the swing phase.

In hemiplegics the strong linkage between quadriceps and plantar flexors prevents the swing and the affected limb is moved forward by other compensatory mechanism.

Hip Joint

Early to midstance: In normals during weight bearing the abductors of that hip prevent the pelvis from sagging on the opposite side along with trunk flexors. The hip extensors work from heel strike to midstance. This short burst of activity reduces just before midstance.

In hemiplegics due to activation of the extensor synergy, the adductors contract in place of abductors and hence there is Trendelenburg sign. Moreover when the adductor spasticity is very severe the affected leg is placed very close to the normal limb or may even cross over interfering grossly with the forward propulsion.

Swing Phase

In normals this begins in late stance and is due to combined effort of muscles, gravitational force and momemtum. EMG studies have shown that the muscle activity level is minimal. The hip flexors, knee flexor and dorsiflexors act to help in adequate ground clearance.

In hemiplegics the extensor synergy does not let go its grip and if does then it is very slowly so that the body moves forward in slow manner. Hip and knee flexion is absent because of plantar flexion at the ankle and retracted pelvis. Thus there is inadequate ground clearance. In the absence of forward rotation of the pelvis and hip flexion the limb is brought forward by circumduction. Occasionally the limb may be dragged behind with the pelvis posterior, hip in external rotation and toes facing laterally.

Assessment

The physiotherapist should be competent in assessment of a patient with stroke to find about the extent and severity of the involvement, to detect the influence of the secondary musculoskeletal changes that will determine the ultimate functional outcome of the patient.

History

The history of the patient in terms of the onset, duration of the illness, progression, associated features, previous treatment and the present status of the patient should be noted.

ON OBSERVATION

Posture: The patients general posture, the attitude of the upper and lower limb, and the facial symmetry should be checked.

Other secondary manifestation like skin changes, presence of edema should be noted.

ON EXAMINATION

Higher function testing: The higher function testing includes assessing the memory, intelligence, consciousness, behavior, orientation and speech.

Cranial nerve testing: The cranial nerve should be assessed for their involvement as their affection may interfere in the rehabilitation process.

Sensory Examination

Evaluation of the sensory involvement gives an indication about the severity of the primary lesion and also determines the extent of improvement in these patients.

The following sensory involvement should be carried out:
- *Superficial:* Crude touch and fine touch
- *Deep:* Pressure, joint position sensation, kinesthetic sensation and vibration sensation.
- *Cortical sensation:* Tactile localization and stereognosis.
- Involvement of only the cortical sensation indicates that the lesion in the sensory cortex area. Involvement of the other sensation indicates an extensive subcortical lesion. Absence of sensory involvement indicates that the lesion is only localized to the motor areas of the brain or a reversible lesion with a good prognosis.

Motor Examination

Tone: The tone of the muscles is tested by fast passive movement to determine the distribution and severity of spasticity. It should be done at all the joints. Usually the muscles exhibit clasp knife type of spasticity. Spasticity may be graded as mild, moderate or severe based upon the restriction to passive movement.

Range of motion should be assessed at each joint. The range may be restricted due to the presence of spasticity, contracture, or adhesion within the joint.

Contracture or deformity: It is necessary to find out the muscles or the group of muscles, which has developed contracture. It should be noted whether the contracture is a mild or severe one.

One should know to distinguish between tightness and spasticity. This is essential because the physiotherapy approach will be different in both of these conditions.

Voluntary Control Testing

The brain appreciates movement performed and not the muscles hence it is very essential that in patients with upper motor neuron involvement the control of the patient for isolated movement at each joint should be checked. Earlier concepts of voluntary control testing comprised of six grades.

Grade 0 — No contraction or flicker or initiation.

Grade II — Flicker of contraction present or initation of movement.

Grade II — Half range of motion in synergy or abnormal pattern.

Grade III— Full range of motion in synergy or abnormal pattern.

Grade IV— Initial half range is performed in isolation and the latter half in pattern.

Grade V — Full range of motion in isolation but goes into pattern when resistance is offered.

Grade VI— Full range of motion in isolation against resistance.

This voluntary control testing should be performed at all the joints and for all the movements. The starting position given to the patient should be either neutral or anti-synergist position and the therapist should ask the patient to perform a specific movement without any other associated movement performed at the same joint or other joint. Presence of contracture or deformity indicates the presence of a mechanical factor and hence should not be considered as a pattern.

However, the (STREAM) scoring of the voluntary movements which is as follows has made the concept of voluntary control testing very simpler.

0 — Unable to perform the test movement through any appreciable range (includes flicker or slight movement).

1 — Able to perform only part of the movement or complete the full movement with marked deviation from normal pattern.

2 — Able to complete the movement in a manner that is comparable to the unaffected side.

Functional Assessment

The assessment of hemiplegic is incomplete without finding the patients level of functional independence. The functional activities should be checked in lying, sitting, and standing posture.

Lying: The activities that need to be assessed are pelvic rotation, bridging, turning, rolling and various reaching out activities.

Sitting: The activities that need to be assessed are weight shifts, turning, bending, lateral bending, as well as functions of upper extremities like eating, brushing, combing, buttoning and reaching out activities. Balance of the patient can be checked by giving perturbation or by making the patient sit on a vestibular ball.

Standing: Static balance, weight shift, turning, and walking should be assessed.

Gait analysis should include observation of whether the patient walks independently, his balance in walking, turning around, and the various gait determinants should be checked for.

Information about various activities for personal hygiene that includes, washing face, bathing, and toilet activities should be taken from the patient.

MANAGEMENT

There are various physiotherapy approaches to the rehabilitation of stroke patient with hemiplegia.

Bobath: This is based on normal movement or neuro-development approach. The main aim is to prevent abnormal movement and adverse plastic adaptations and to facilitate normal movement and subsequent plastic changes (Bobath 1990).

Brunstorn (1970): He makes use of abnormal synergies and incorporate them into functional activities.

Conductive education (Peto): This was developed by Cotton and Kinsman (1983). The patient is encouraged to verbalize the activities as they perform them. This focuses on function.

Johnstone (1989): Follows developmental sequence, i.e. focussing on proximal stability. It makes use of orally inflated pressure splints.

Motor relearning program: This was described by Carr-Shepherd in the year 1987. This training of motor control is based on an understanding of kinematics and kinetics of normal movement, motor control process and motor learning.

Proprioceptive neuromuscular facilitation (PNF): This was developed by Knott and Voss in the year 1968. To maximize sensory stimuli on the pool of AHC in order to stimulate purposeful muscle contraction.

Roods: This was first practiced by Stock and Meyer in the year 1966. This was mainly done to achieve purposeful muscular contraction by stimulating the skin through facilitating strokes on the skin. The stimulus given through the skin can have facilitatory and inhibitory effects.

Recent studies have shown that no single treatment can produce the desired response in different patients and that different therapist relies on different methods in treating hemiplegia. Thus one specific technique alone may be inadequate to produce the beneficial effect in stroke patient. The author uses an integrated approach using, Bobath, Burnstorm, Motor relearning, Roods,PNF and other form of sensory integration in treating patient with hemiplegia. The combination of treatment used differs from patient to patient.

The management of hemiplegia is different based upon the stage of the hemiplegic patient.

Acute Stage

The goals of the treatment in acute stage are:
a. Prevent ignorance or unawareness of the hemiplegic side.
b. Decrease the tendency to develop synergy in the chronic stage.
c. Prevention of any joint restriction or stiffness.
d. Prevention of complications due to immobilization like chest complication, deconditioning of the bone and muscles, etc.
e. Early weight bearing.
f. Psychological counselling.
g. Education to the family.
   These goals can be achieved through the following treatment.

Arrangement of the Patient's Room (Fig. 2.3)

Due to the lesion the patient suffers from sensory deprivation that leads to neglect of the hemiplegic side which can be greatly influenced by the patient's head position. Hence all the forms of the stimulus like the entrance to the room, the relatives, television, etc. should be present on the hemiplegic side so that the patient is forced to turn to that side which will stimulate awareness of the hemiplegic side.

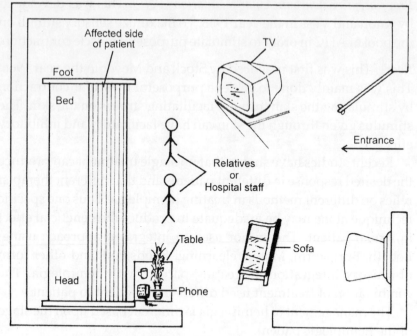

Fig. 2.3: Arrangement of the room for stroke patient

Positioning (Figs 2.4 to 2.6)

Positioning of the patient in an appropriate way is essential to control the development of spasticity and to help in faster improvement in the later stages. Preferably the patient is positioned sidelying and supine generally avoided.

On the affected side: The shoulder should be protracted and flexed. The elbow and the wrist should be extended. The forearm should be supinated. The pelvis should be in protracted position. The hip and knee should be in slight flexion and the ankle should be in neutral position.

On the sound side: The arm should be rested on the pillow kept in front of the patient. The shoulder girdle should be kept in protraction and slight elevation. The shoulder is kept in slight abduction and flexion with the elbow and wrist in extension position. The forearm should be in supine position. The pelvis should be kept in protraction. The hip should be slightly abducted and flexed. The knee should be slightly flexed and the ankle should be in neutral position.

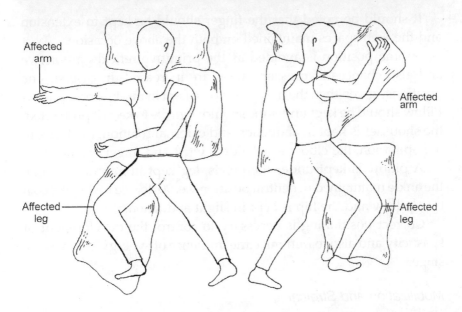

Fig. 2.4: Lying on affected side   **Fig. 2.5:** Lying on unaffected side

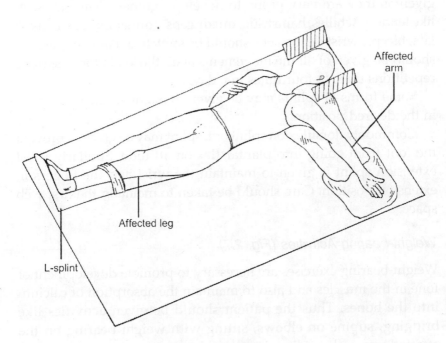

Fig. 2.6: Lying in supine position

It should be noted that the finger should be kept in extension and the web spaces maintained on both the above occasion.

Supine position is avoided as the primitive reflexes are active and also chances of pressure sores are increased. In case supine position is given then the head should be kept in midline on a pillow. Pillow should be kept under the shoulder girdle to keep it protracted, the shoulder is kept in abduction and external rotation, the forearm in supination, the elbow is extended, wrist and finger extended.

A pillow is kept under the pelvis, leg kept in neutral rotation, the ankle maintained in neutral position, i.e. 90 degree of dorsiflexion by a pillow and the hip is kept in slight abduction.

Correct positioning is necessary to control the development of spasticity and also to minimize the influence of synergy in spasticity stage.

Mobilization and Stretching

During flaccid stage mobilization in the form of gentle passive exercises and stretching of various biarticular muscles should be given as they are very prone to develop tightness. Thus muscles like tendon Achilles, hamstring, quadriceps, adductors, tensor fascia lata, biceps, wrist flexors, etc. should be stretched. Passive exercises should be given of all the movements at all the joints for at least 10 repetitions three to four times in a day.

Some forms of splints may be given to maintain the body parts in the desired position.

Commonly dorsiflexion splint or L splint may be given to prevent the foot from going into plantar flexion attitude. Similarly wrist extension splint is given to maintain the wrist and the fingers in extension position. Care should be taken to maintain the first web space.

Weight-bearing Activities (Fig. 2.7)

Weight-bearing exercises are necessary to promote development of tone in the muscles and also to maintain the absorption of calcium into the bones. Thus the patient should be given activities like bridging, supine on elbows, sitting with weight bearing on the affected arm, and standing should be given as soon as possible within the limitation of the patient's general medical status.

Subluxation of the glenohumeral joint is a very common complication in stroke patient, which can be prevented by proper

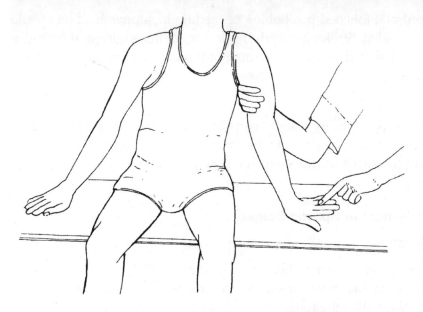

Fig. 2.7: Weight-bearing through affected upper limb

positioning and handling. Some form of support may be given to prevent distraction of the joint when the patient assumes an erect position. Generally a shoulder sling or Bobath splint is given to prevent this complication. Skillful taping also helps in preventing the subluxation very effectively and in addition also gives room for free movement. It also gives a tactile feedback which helps in faster development of tone in the shoulder muscles. Weight bearing exercises for the involved upper limb has also been found to be beneficial in preventing this. Shoulder sling is usually avoided as it facilitated the hemiplegic attitude, which the patient may develop in later stages.

Chest Physiotherapy

Chest physiotherapy in the form of inspiratory breathing exercises should be given to maintain the lung compliance and to prevent any chances of secretion accumulation. In cases of necessity nebulization or postural drainage can be given.

Oropharyngeal Retraining

Swallowing difficulty, which the patient has, can be counteracted by giving a proper positioning and by developing proper head control. Slouched positioning or feeding in supine position should be avoided. Stroking over the neck area, ice massaging of the tongue, stimulating lip closure are some of the various techniques that are used to facilitate swallowing.

Counseling

As the patients are usually very depressed, the therapist should try and motivate the patient. The therapist should have a very cheerful and confident attitude, which will help the patient in keeping a high moral.

Treatment in Spastic Stages

Spasticity

It is always better to keep the spasticity under control. In case of spasticity the therapist should try to achieve the following aims:
- Normalize the tone.
- Development of normal functional pattern.
- Prevention of contracture and deformity.
- Train the patient to be functionally independent.
- Achieve highest possible physical security for the patient.

Normalization of the tone can be achieved by reducing the tone of the spastic muscles and simultaneously strengthening the weak antagonist muscles. Spasticity in the muscles can be reduced by the following methods:
- Gentle rhythmic passive movement.
- Sustained gradual stretching either manually or by using splints.
- Prolonged icing over the spastic muscle bulk for about 15 to 20 minutes. Studies have shown that prolonged icing and sustained stretching are equally effective in inhibiting spasticity.
- Faradic stimulation to the weak antagonist muscles can reduce the spasticity of the agonist muscle by the principle of reciprocal inhibition. However, this should be given only when the antagonist muscle is not active voluntarily.
- Reflex inhibiting postures or pattern. Infact, almost all the exercises given in the stage of spasticity are on the basis of reflex inhibiting pattern and postures.
- Biofeedback : This can be used to relax spastic muscle as well as to activate its antagonist.

Activities in Spastic Stage

Exercises in Lying (Figs 2.8A to L)

- *Scapular movement:* The patient scapula should be mobilized passively and also the patient should be asked to perform protraction and elevation movement of the scapula.
- *Touching the opposite shoulder:* The patient is trained to take his arm from extension, abduction and external rotation position toward his opposite shoulder into flexion, adduction, supination and external rotation.
- *Touching the head:* The patient is trained to touch the head by maintaining external rotation and supination.

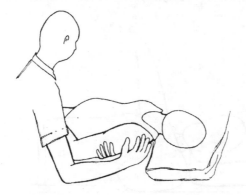

Fig. 2.8A: Guiding shoulder girdle movement

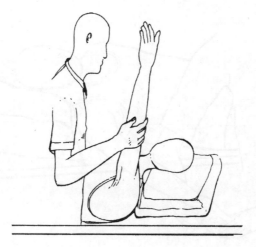

Fig. 2.8B: Protraction-retraction of shoulder girdle

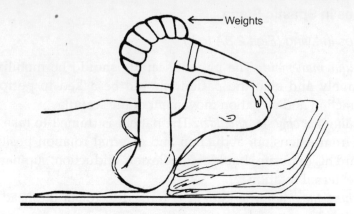

Fig. 2.8C: Developing shoulder control by balancing weight

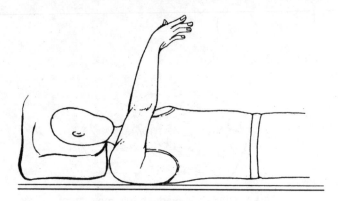

Fig. 2.8D: Holding arm in space

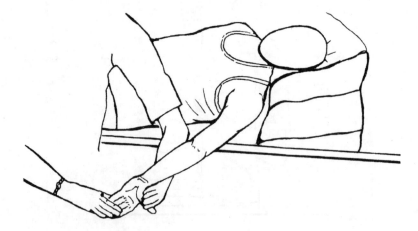

Fig. 2.8E: Extension abduction to flexion adduction pattern

- The therapist maintains the hand in extension of the fingers with the thumb in abducted position and then she moves the hand into abduction and elevation maintaining the elbow in extension. This exercise can be progressed to active as the patient learns to control the movement.
- Elbow extension with shoulder in 90 degree of flexion.
- The patient is then trained to maintain the arm in space in different directions. This exercise will help the patient in developing good control of the upper limbs and also increases the proximal fixation.
- *Bridging:* Bridging should be done by weight bearing on the affected limb only. The therapist maintains the normal limb in flexion and encourages weight bearing through the hemiplegic lower extremities.

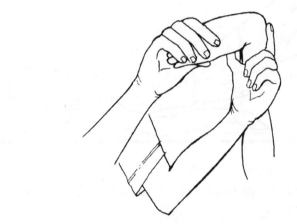

Fig. 2.8F: Correct way of holding hand to inhibit long flexor spasticity

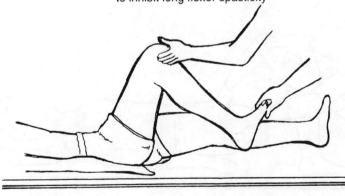

Fig. 2.8G: Hip-knee extension with ankle dorsiflexion

- *Unilateral rotation of the pelvis:* The patient performs hip-knee flexion of the affected lower limb and then rotated the pelvis to the opposite side. The patient tries to maintain this posture so that the spasticity of the trunk is inhibited. This exercise also help in encouraging forward rotation of the pelvis and correcting pelvic retraction.
- The patient is encouraged to perform flexion adduction and extension abduction pattern of the lower limb keeping the knee in extension position throughout.
- The affected lower limb is kept in abduction at the edge of the plinth such that the knee is in flexion. In this position the patient is encouraged to perform knee extension and flexion without

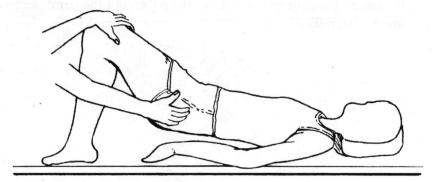

Fig. 2.8H: Bridging activity to improve pelvic control

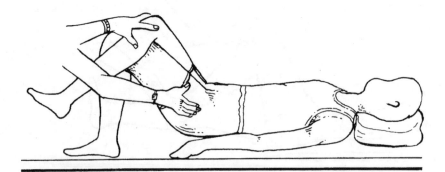

Fig. 2.8I: Bridging by taking weight on the affected lower limb

any addition of flexion also ensures the line that system will ... ...

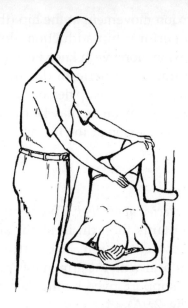

Fig. 2.8J: Pelvic rotation with hip knee flexion to inhibit trunk spasticity

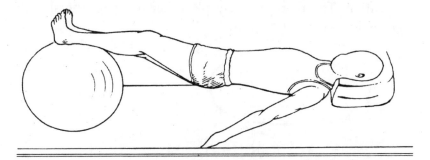

Fig. 2.8K: Bridging on vestibular ball to improve pelvic control

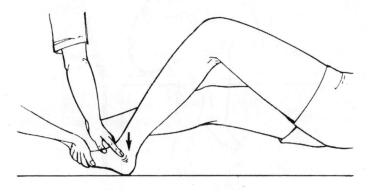

Fig. 2.8L: Facilitating dorsiflexion of foot

any adduction or flexion movement at the hip (the patient will have a tendency to perform hip adduction along with knee extension and hip flexion along with knee flexion).

- The patient may be trained to perform dorsiflexion with hip extension and plantar flexion with hip flexion. In case the patient is unable to perform dorsiflexion he may be trained to do with hip-knee flexion and the flexion at the hip and knee gradually reduced.

Exercises in Sitting

- *Weight bearing on the affected upper limb:* The therapist sits behind the patient and maintains the arm in slight abduction and extension with elbow extension. The patient should be encouraged to weight bear with the arm in this position. As the patient improves the support given by the therapist should be gradually reduced (Fig. 2.9A).
- *Shoulder shrugs:* This exercises help the patient to achieve scapular elevation. The therapist may place her hand on the shoulder girdle to give a tactile input.

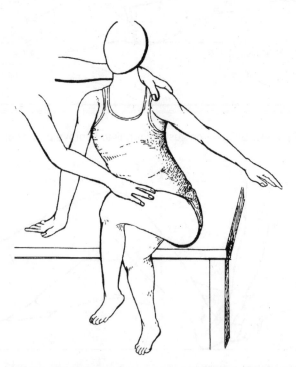

Fig. 2.9A: Facilitating weight transmission through affected side

- *Touching the opposite shoulder and placing the hand on the sacrum:* The patient is trained to touch the opposite shoulder in supination and then take it behind the back as far across as possible to the opposite side.
- *In sitting position some exercises for the hand can be given emphasizing more on the extension components.* Visual feed back exercises like holding a paper glass with water in it such that the water level should not increase or holding a clay mould without causing hand impression are some of the ways to train control of the hand.
- *Supination pronation* keeping the elbow flexed at 90 degrees.
- *Knee extension and flexion of the knee*: The patient should be asked to flex the knee by taking the foot as much as possible below the chair and then straightening it.
- *Getting up*: The patient is trained to perform getting up by moving the foot closer to the chair, bending forward, holding the hand rest and then getting up.
- *Vestibular exercises*: The patient may be made to sit on the vestibular ball to improve the balance and also normalize the tone of the trunk. Vestibular ball may be used to exercise the upper extremities mainly to achieve control at the proximal joint and facilitate extension of the fingers through stimulation of the proprioceptors at all the joints of the upper limb (Fig. 2.9B).

Exercises in Standing

In standing the patient is trained to achieve static balance by giving perturbation or by making the person stand on a wobble board or tilt board. Balance should also be trained in step stance. The patient is trained to shift weight alternately on both the lower limbs. Standing should be encouraged by keeping the affected leg slightly behind the normal leg to facilitate more weight-bearing on that side (Fig. 2.10).

Dynamic balance can be trained in standing by teaching various reaching out activities and also by teaching the patient rotation of the trunk and forward bending exercises. These exercises also help in development of automatic adaptation of the muscles which is important for performance of many activities. The patient balance should be trained for anticipatory and automatic response.

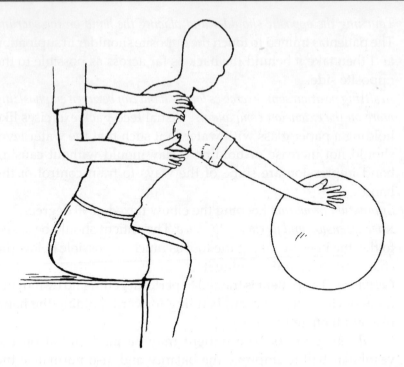

Fig. 2.9B: Approximation exercise for upper limb on vestibular ball. The patient can also be asked to move the ball with affected arm to develop control

The following exercises may be given in standing:
- The therapist stands behind the patient and hold the pelvis such that the affected pelvis is kept in protraction. The patient is then encouraged to place the affected leg forward and then take it back. This is repeated for 10 times. Similarly the patient is encouraged to place the affected leg to the sides (abduction) and then come to the neutral position for ten times. This activities help the patient during swing phase of the gait cycle.
- In the same position, the therapist trains the patient to take weight on the affected leg and place the normal leg forward and then back. This is repeated ten times. Similarly abduction movement can also be trained for 10 times. This activity encourages proper weight bearing of the affected limb.
- Symmetrical throwing activities should be encouraged to increase the balance reaction and also to increase the stability limit which will help the patient in proper postural control.
- Unilateral stance on the affected leg should be given to the patient which will facilitate isometric work of the abductors to prevent Trendeleburg's sign.

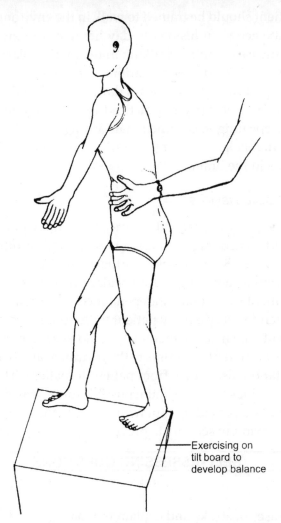

Exercising on
tilt board to
develop balance

Fig. 2.10: Tilt board exercises for improving balance and control of lower limb

Once the patient is comfortably doing the above exercises then he may be trained to walk in between the parallel bars in a near normal gait pattern. Side walking and backward walking should also be given. Then progressed to walking unaided on the level ground.

Treadmill training or using a static cycle to train the gait in hemiplegic patient, especially in the early stages, has been found to improve the gait pattern to a remarkable extent. Treadmill walking with partial weight supporting harness have been useful in rehabilitating gait in hemiplegics.

The patient should be trained to walk in the environment which he will come across in his day-to-day life like walking on uneven surface, staircase climbing, walking in the market place, etc.

Once the patient develops various components of movement available to perform his activities of daily living the basic functional activities should be directly practiced to gain independency and accuracy. Repeating each functional task again and again over a period of times helps in faster learning of those task by formation of the engrams in the brain.

Use of Assistive Devices

Based on the pathological and security limit of the patient, he may or may not be encouraged to use a walking aid or other forms of assistive devices. Some forms of orthosis like AFO or knee brace may be given in cases of gross muscular imbalance that interferes with the patient's functional independence. Cane or a walking stick may be given for very elderly patient with poor balance reaction.

One point which all the therapist should keep in mind is that the patient show different responses to the treatment and hence the goal of rehabilitation also varies from patient to patient. The main aim should be to achieve the maximum possible functional independence for a patient and providing him with measure that will help him in achieving maximum security to prevent any further damage to him.

SELF-ASSESSING QUESTIONS

Long Eassy

- Give causes of stroke and explain the management.
- Describe the circle of Willis and give its importance.
- Explain the blood supply to the brain and describe various stroke syndromes.
- Explain the assessment of patient with stroke.
- Discuss the principle of assessment of a 60 years old stroke patient with hemiplegia of non-dominant side.
- Explain the clinical presentation of a stroke patient.
- Describe the various methods of functional retraining for the various tasks of the upper limb like eating, reaching out, weight-bearing.
- Describe various techniques of rehabilitating a hemiplegic gait

- Describe the principles of underlying physiotherapy management of stroke patient.
- Explain the significance of reflex inhibiting position and pattern in treatment of stroke.
- Physiotherapy role in flaccid stage of stroke.

Short Eassy

- Circle of Willis.
- Management of spastic hand.
- Perceptual disorders in stroke.
- Motor abnormality in stroke.
- Management of spastic foot.
- Management of spasticity.
- Hemiplegic gait.
- Exercises to improve gait in hemiplegia.
- Exercises to improve various hand functions.
- Voluntary control testing.

Short Answers

- What is apraxia?
- What is agnosia and its types?
- Types of apraxia.
- What is Gerstmann's syndrome?
- Define autotopagnosia?
- What is somatognosia?
- Aphasia and its types.
- What is hemianopia?
- Principles of rood approach.
- What is motor relearning?
- What is reflex inhibiting pattern?
- Difference between associated reaction and associated movements.

3

Incoordination

Before knowing incoordination one should know how a coordinated movement appear so that it is very easy to detect any abnormality that may be noted in it. Coordinated movements are those that appear to be smooth, accurate and purposeful, is brought about by the integrated action of many muscles, superimposed upon a basis of efficient postural activity. Coordinated movements are characterized by appropriate speed, distance, direction, rhythm and muscle tension.

Incoordination and coordination deficit are general terms used to describe abnormal motor function characterized by awkward, extraneous, uneven or inaccurate movements.

The performance of movement in a coordinated manner also depends upon the formation of engram in the brain. Engram represents neurological organization of a preprogrammed patterns of muscular activity. Once the engram is formed each time it is excited it automatically produces same pattern. Engram is dependent upon control that is conscious activation of an individual muscle or the conscious initiation of a preprogrammed engram. In order to have a smooth coordinated movement, nervous control is very much essential which operates at six main levels as follows.

CEREBELLUM

It is the largest part of the hindbrain that lies posterior to the pons and the medulla oblongata in the posterior cranial fossa. It is somewhat ovoid in shape and constricted in the median part. It consists of two cerebellar hemispheres which are joined by a narrow median vermis. Each hemisphere is connected to three parts of the brainstem by way of three cerebellar peduncles. The cerebellum is divided into three main lobes anterior, posterior and flocculonodular by deep transverse fissures. Longitudinally, besides the vermis lies the intermediate zone of the hemisphere and laterally lies the lateral zone of the hemisphere.

Phylogenetically the cerebellum is divided into

- Archicerebellum made of flocculonodular part is the oldest part of the cerebellum and is associated with the vestibular system.
- Neocerebellum made up of posterior lobe and is associated with fine voluntary movement.
- Paleocerebellum composed of anterior lobe, uvula and pyramid of vermis is functionally related to gross movements of the head and body.

Internally the cerebellum is composed of grey matter and white matter. The gray matter forms the cortex of the cerebellum and is situated within the cerebellum as cerebellar nuclei. The cortex of the cerebellum is formed of three layers namely the molecular layer, the purkinge cell layer and the granular layer. The cerebellar nuclei are dentate, emboliform, globose and fastigial.

The white matter of the cerebellum consists of intrinsic fibers, which do not leave the cerebellum, but connects its different parts, the afferent fibres and the efferent fibers. The afferent fibers are corticopontocerebellar pathway, olivocerebellar, vestibulocerebellar and reticulocerebellar fibers. The efferent fibers from the cerebellum go to the medulla, pons, thalamus, cortex, and basal ganglia (Fig. 3.1).

In fact, the word cerebellum means "little brain" and yet this region of brain contains more neurons than all the rest of the brain put together. This little brain also has a large role in the motor control and motor learning. The main function of the cerebellum however is coordination of motor activity, equilibrium and muscle tone.

The cerebellum works mainly as comparator and error correcting mechanism. The cerebellum compares the commands for movement transmitted from the motor cortex with the actual motor performance of the body segments. This occurs by a comparison of information received from the cortex with the information obtained from peripheral feed back mechanism. The motor cortex and brainstem motor structures provide the commands for the intended motor response. Peripheral feedback during the motor response is provided by muscle spindles, golgi tendon organs, joint and cutaneous receptors, the vestibular apparatus and the eyes and ears.

If the input from the feedback system does not compare appropriately (that is the movement that deviates from the intended

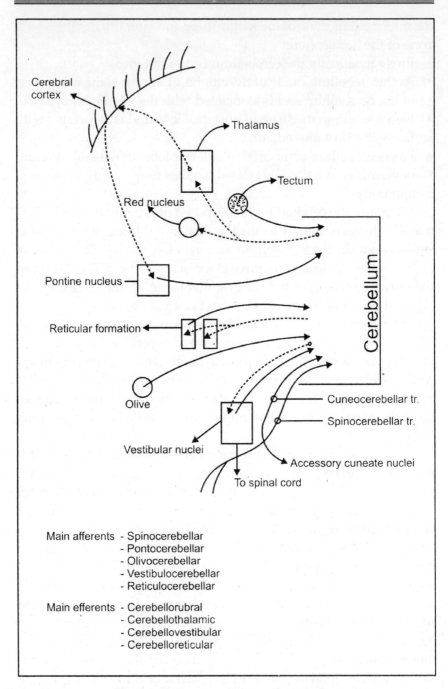

Cerebral cortex

Thalamus

Tectum

Red nucleus

Pontine nucleus

Reticular formation

Olive

Cerebellum

Cuneocerebellar tr.

Spinocerebellar tr.

Vestibular nuclei

Accessory cuneate nuclei

To spinal cord

Main afferents - Spinocerebellar
               - Pontocerebellar
               - Olivocerebellar
               - Vestibulocerebellar
               - Reticulocerebellar

Main efferents - Cerebellorubral
               - Cerebellothalamic
               - Cerebellovestibular
               - Cerebelloreticular

Fig. 3.1: Various connections of cerebellum

command), the cerebellum supplies a corrective influence. This is achieved by corrective signals sent to the cortex which via motor pathway modifies or corrects the ongoing movement. This error correction is referred to as a closed loop system. Stereotypical movements (gait activity) and rapid short duration movements which do not allow sufficient time for feedback to occur are controlled by an open loop system.

The cerebellum also helps in planning of sequential movements. The plan of sequential movement is transmitted from the sensory and premotor areas of the cortex to the lateral zone of the cerebellar hemisphere. A two-way traffic is essential for transfer from one movement to the other movement. Timing of movement is also brought about by the lateral zone of the cerebellar hemisphere.

Impairments in Cerebellar Disease

Dysmetria

It is inability to accurately judge the direction, distance, extent, force and timing of limb movement. Clinically it is manifested as past pointing whenever the patient tries to touch an object. Speed of the movement is somewhat slow and there is irregularity during both acceleration and deceleration of movement. A lack of programmed deceleration was thought to be responsible for dysmetria. The dampening circuit in the cerebellum is responsible for halting any limb movement and this function is lost in cerebellar dysfunction.

Movement Decomposition

As the patient with cerebellar lesion cannot perform a particular movement in a single pattern at a time, he breaks the movement into its various component parts and performs one by one. This is called as movement decomposition. The abnormal timing and duration of contraction and relaxation of muscle has also been thought of contributing to the decomposition of movement. In monkeys however it is shown that cooling the dentate nucleus decomposes the movement.

Ataxia

It is a classical sign of cerebellar dysfunction. It represents combined influence of dysmetria and movement decomposition on gait, posture, and pattern of movement in cerebellar dysfunction. The ataxic manifestations are typically seen in the gait of the patient. The cerebellum has anatomical connections, which influence the normal pattern of locomotion. The cerebellum receives information about the gait from the spinal cord and it sends its control indirectly via the rubrospinal, reticulospinal and vestibulospinal tracts. This circuit ensures a very rhythmical smooth locomotion that is seen under normal circumstances. Ataxic movement can be seen in the limbs or trunk but is very evident when the patient walks. Due to cerebellar lesion the gait becomes typical ataxic in which there is uneven step length, wide base and arrhythmic.

If the central cerebellar structures like vermis or flocculo-nodular lobe are involved then the ataxia involves central structures of the body and is very apparent when the patient is standing, sitting or walking. This is called as central ataxia or truncal. Lesser degree of central ataxia can be provoked by making the patient do tandem walking, heel–toe walking. There will be titubation of head in which the head oscillates in anteroposterior manner.

Rebound Phenomenon

This occurs due to loss of cerebellar component of stretch reflex. Normally cerebellum instantaneously adds a large amount of additional feedback support to the spinal cord stretch reflex mechanism whenever a portion of the body begins to move unexpectedly in an unwilled direction. Clinically, it can be tested by suddenly removing a resisting force from an isometrically contracting limb. In a normal person the limb will not change position. In contrast the limb of a person with a cerebellar lesion will move abruptly as if still opposing the resistance thus lacking control.

Hypotonicity

It refers to decrease in the normal resistance offered by the muscle to passive movement or palpation. This is due to depression of the excitatory signals from the deep nuclei of the cerebellum to the regions of the brain that excites the alpha and gamma motor neuron. When the limb is suddenly dropped the extremity will fall rapidly without correcting itself. Hypotonicity has been noted more in acute lesions than in chronic cases. It is noted in experimental animals that in cerebellar hypotonicity there is depression of fusimotor efferent and spindle afferent activity. With passage of time the fusimotor activity returns and the hypotonia disappears. The presence of hypotonicity more in acute lesion could be related to the above mechanisms.

Pendular Reflexes

The deep tendon reflexes are not lost but behaves in a pendular fashion after the initial contraction of the muscle. This is due to the lack of dampening function of the cerebellum hence after initial contraction, the limb fall by its own weight and momentarily oscillates in a pendular manner and stops after some time. Presence of hypotonicity further makes the pendular jerk more obvious.

Dysdiadocokinesia

The patient has difficulty in performing rapid alternating movements. Inability to perform these movements is called as adiadochokinesia. The most useful tests are in which the patient is asked to tap the foot or hand on the floor. Also the patient will not be able to perform rapid supination and pronation. In ADL, the patient finds activities such as brushing the teeth, polishing the shoe, cutting vegetables, etc. difficult to perform. Dysdiadochokinesia is related to dysmetria in that both result from the inappropriate timing of muscle activity. The inability to stop the activity is termed as dysmetria whereas inability to reverse the direction of movement at the same speed indicates adiadochokinesia. If he performs with difficulty then it is called dysdiadochokinesia.

Tremor

Intentional tremor is noted in cerebellar lesions. In intentional tremor the hand oscillates back and forth as the patients try to touch their nose or the heel oscillates as they attempt to slide it down the opposite shin. The tremor has a frequency of 3 to 5 Hz and is typically enhanced during the termination of a goal directed movement. It occurs due to cerebellar overshoot and failure in the dampening. The dentate nucleus has been found to inhibit this abnormal oscillatory movement in experimental studies.

Postural tremor that occurs when the patient tries to maintain the normal erect posture may be noted in cerebellar dysfunction although it may not be as frequent as intentional tremor. The postural tremor could be possibly due to disruption of proprioceptive feedback loops.

A head tremor of moderate speed (3-4/sec) in anteroposterior direction often accompanies midline cerebellar lesion like that of damage to the vermis.

Ocular Disturbances

This occurs due to lesion of the posterior vermis and the flocculo-nodular lobe. Voluntary gaze is accomplished by a series of jerky movements, which is called as saccadic dysmetria. On attempted fixation of vision the eyes may overshoot the target and then oscillate through several cycles until pressure fixation is attained. Nystagmus may not be an essential feature of cerebellar lesion. The common type of nystagmus is called as Gaze-paretic nystagmus in which there is inability to hold eccentric position of gaze resulting in need to make repetitive saccades to look eccentrically. Other nystagmus that may be seen are Down beat nystagmus and Rebound nystagmus. Ocular flutter may be noted in some patients in which there is occasional burst of very rapid to and fro flutter like horizontal oscillation around the point of fixation.

Speech Disturbance

Disturbance in speech that is seen in cerebellar syndrome is termed as dysarthria. This can be of two forms one in which there is simple, slow, slurring of speech and the other in which there is scanned speech. Words are broken into individual syllables. The pronunciation is slow, accents are misplaced and the pauses may be inappropriately short or long. The patient may also have explosive speech or staccato speech in which the syllables may be uttered with less or more force. The voice can become invariant in pitch and loudness. However the grammar or word selection is not altered.

Balance and Equilibrium

The cerebellum is a vital structure in maintenance of the upright posture. Lesion of the cerebellum involving the vestibulocerebellum or the fastigial nucleus results in postural sway and poor equilibrium reactions which cannot be controlled by use of visual feedback. The person with cerebellar dysfunction does not modify the reflex even with repeated presentations of the appropriate stimulus.

Asthenia

Patient with cerebellar lesion can have a state of generalized weakness called as asthenia. The strength of the involved side may be reduced by about 50 percent in unilateral injury to the cerebellum. The mechanism is not clear. Theoretically speaking it could be due to loss of cerebellar facilitation to the motor cortex which in turn reduce the activity of spinal motor neurons during voluntary movement. Also deconditioning of the muscles due to reduced activity could be contributory factor in chronic cases.

Basal Ganglia

The basal ganglia include caudate nucleus, putamen and globus pallidus that is situated in the base of the cerebral cortex. Basal ganglia lesions by virtue of causing symptoms like Rigidity, Bradykinesia, Tremors can make the movement appear incoordinated. Basal ganglia lesions also cause certain movement disorders like chorea, athetosis, hemiballismus which further make the movement incoordinated. The syndromes, which are associated with clinical features of basal ganglia lesions are Parkinson's disease, Wilson's disease and Hungtinton's chorea. Parkinson's disease is explained in detail in the Chapter 5 "Parkinsonism".

Upper Motor Neuron (Motor Cortex)

Initiation center exists in the brainstem that alerts the cerebral cortex that in turn is responsible for planning the pattern of movement.

The major problem of the type of lesion is spasticity. The spasticity causes development of abnormal movement patterns which are not significant for functional activities. These movements appear to be incoordinated. The mode of management is to first break the abnormal pattern of movement that has set in and then go for precision of movement. For instance in hemiplegia the upper extremity remains in flexion at the shoulder, elbow flexion, wrist flexion with forearm across the chest. For ADL like eating it is necessary to have wrist extension and hence the first two components which is the shoulder and elbow flexion are maintained while the patient is asked to do wrist extension in the initial range, intermediate range as well as in the end range. The hold of the therapist should never be on the spastic muscle but on the opposite muscles.

Lower Motor Neuron

It is not a classical incoordination. Lower motor neuron lesions are seen in diseases like neuropathies, myopathies or PNI. Here all other factors are normal but the right impulses don't reach the muscle hence there is no contraction of the muscle. Since the actual muscle don't have the power the patient uses other muscles to perform trick movements which appear to be jerky and may be called incoordinated.

Dorsal Columns

The dorsal columns are necessary for mediating proprioceptive signals from the muscles and joint receptors to the higher centers. Proprioceptive information is necessary to make one aware of the position of the body parts in space as well as the various movements taking place in the body segments. Hence the dorsal column plays a very important role in coordinating movements as well as maintenance of normal posture. Lack of proprioceptive information to the cerebellum will make a person unaware of his joint position as well as movement. The various adjustments, adaptation and judgement that is necessary for any activity is lost due to lack of proprioceptive signals and these make the movement very incoordinated. In fact whenever the proprioceptive signals are lost the patient tries to substitute for its loss by using the visual feedback to assist him in various movements and postural control. It may serve the purpose partially but the functions become very inefficient. This kind of symptoms may be seen in neurosyphilis of the spinal cord (*Tabes dorsalis*).

Friedreich's Ataxia

Friedreich's ataxia is an early onset type of hereditary spino-cerebellar ataxia that is progressive in nature. It is due to involvement of the spinocerebellar tract which impairs the sensory component of the cerebellum thereby producing ataxia. In most of the cases the onset is well within the tenth year. Ataxia of the gait is nearly always the initial symptom. The disease progresses so rapidly that within 5 years of onset the patient's walking ability may be totally lost. Initially the patient has difficulty in standing steadily and in running. The hand becomes clumpsy month or year after the gait disorder and this is followed by dysarthria. The patient develops kyphoscoliosis of the spine. The foot has a typical pes cavus with hammer toes. All the tests for sensory ataxia will be positive in Friedriech's ataxia. The speech is slow, slurred, explosive and incomprehensible. Breathing, speaking, swallowing, and laughing may be so incoordinated that the patient nearly chokes while speaking. The tendon reflexes gets abolished. Plantar response are extensor and flexor spasm may occur even with complete loss of tendon reflex indicating that the areflexia is sensory in origin. Cardiomyopathy and respiratory disorders may be seen in the later stages.

Although many clinical manifestations of tabes dorsalis and Friedreich's ataxia are similar but they are two different types of sensory ataxia observed. The physiotherapy management is same for both these disorders.

Tests for Incoordination

Non-Equilibrium Coordination Tests

- *Finger to nose:* The shoulder is abducted to 90 degree with the elbow extended. The patient is asked to bring the tip of the index finger to the tip of the nose.
- *Finger to therapist finger:* The patient and the therapist sit opposite to each other, the therapist's index finger is held in front of the patient, the patient is asked to touch the tip of the index finger to the therapist's index finger. The position of the therapist finger may be altered during testing to assess ability to change the distance, direction and force of movement.
- *Finger to finger:* Both shoulders are abducted to 90th degree with the elbow extended, the patient is asked to bring both the hand towards the midline and approximate the index fingers from opposing hands.
- *Alternate nose to finger:* The patient alternately touches the tip of the nose and the tip of the therapist's finger with the index finger.
- *Pronation and supination:* With elbow flexed to 90 degree and held close to body, the patient alternately turns the palm up and down. This can be done with shoulder flexed to 90 degree and elbow extended. This test help's in identifying dysdiadochokinesis.
- *Hand or finger tapping:* With the elbow flexed and forearm pronated the patient may be asked to tap the hand or finger on the knee.

- *Tapping foot:* The patient is asked to tap the ball of one foot on the floor without raising the knee. The heel maintains contact with the floor.
- *Alternate heel to knee, heel to toe:* The patient is in supine position. The patient is asked to touch the knee and big toe alternately with the heel of the opposite extremity.
- *Heel on shin:* From a supine position, the heel of one foot is slided up and down the shin of the opposite lower extremity.
- *Drawing a circle:* The patient draws an imaginary circle in the air with either upper or lower extremity (a table or floor may also be used).

Equilibrium Coordination Tests

- Standing in a normal comfortable posture
- Standing with feet together (narrow base of support)
- Standing with one foot exactly infront of the other in tandem position (toe of one foot touching heel of opposite foot)
- Standing on one foot
- Arm position may be altered in each of the above postures (that is arm at sides, over head, hands on waist)
- Displace balance unexpectedly (while carefully guarding patient)
- Standing and then alternate between forward trunk flexion and return to neutral
- Standing with trunk laterally flexed to each side
- Standing to test the ability to maintain an upright posture without visual feedback. This is referred to as negative Rhomberg's sign
- Standing in tandem position from eyes open to eyes closed (sharpened Rhomberg)
- Tandem walking: Walking by placing the heel of one foot directly in front of the toe of the opposite foot
- Walking along a straight line or place feet on floor markers while walking
- Walk side ways, backward, cross-stepping
- March in place
- Stop and start abruptly while walking
- Walk in a circle or alternate direction
- Walk on heels or toes.

Management

The management of ataxia differs based upon the causative factors, logistically speaking ataxia can either occur due to cerebellar dysfunction or due to loss of sensory information to the cerebellum. Thus the management of cerebellar ataxia differs slightly from the ones caused due to sensory impairment.

Certain principles need to be applied while treating cases of ataxia which are as follows:

- Intense concentration of the patient
- Active participation of the patient should be encouraged rather than making the treatment program passive
- Frequent rest period needs to be given to prevent fatigue
- The training room should be quiet to avoid any distraction that can aggravate ataxia
- Patient should be always relaxed and should be given a comfortable as well as properly supported position.
- Repetition of task or sequence of task is very important for recovery
- The guidance given by the therapist holds a very important significance in the treatment.

Factors which has a tendency to increase incoordination should be always discouraged. These factors are strong efforts, insecurity, excitement, strong emotions, pain fatigue.

Certain important goals towards which the physiotherapist can work with the patient are:

- Regulate the limb movements accurately during activities
- Develop postural stability and balance
- Improve the tone of the muscle
- Functional transfers and gait.

Certain factors like strong efforts, insecurity, excitement, pain, fatigue and strong emotions tend to increase incoordination hence these factors should be kept to the minimum while treating patient with incoordination.

While exercising patients with incoordination one should always progress from exercises done at a lower center of gravity to exercises that is done at a higher center of gravity. This consideration is necessary to prevent any chances of fear or insecurity that may interfere in the rehabilitation program.

Various functional activities of the patient can be achieved by giving the following exercises to the patient.

Head and Trunk Control (Fig. 3.2A)

Having a good head and trunk control is a prerequisite to sitting and standing. Most of our ADL activities are done in either of these postures and thus they form an important background against which various significant activities are performed. Patient with poor head control can be treated prone with one or two pillows under the chest of the patient (even a wedge can be used for this purpose). Prone on elbow is another position that can be considered to stimulate proper head control in these patients. Facilitation of neck extensors and shoulder girdle retractors can be achieved by using techniques like brisk stroking, quick stretch or vibration given directly on the muscle bulk. In sitting position one can even use technique of joint approximation or rhythmic stabilization in order to bring about contraction of the neck muscle that in turn can stabilize the neck. Biofeed back can also be tried out to facilitate contraction of postural muscles of the neck and trunk. Good trunk control can be achieved by giving activities like prone on elbow, prone on hand, on all fours, bridging, trunk rotations, etc. Putting the patient prone on vestibular ball also helps in developing control of the trunk extensors. Side sitting by taking weight alternately on both the hands also stimulates trunk stabilization.

Getting up from Lying to Sitting Position

Generally it is noted that an ataxic patient has a tendency to log roll rather than to perform segmental rolling. This tendency should be inhibited and the patient should be encouraged to perform segmental

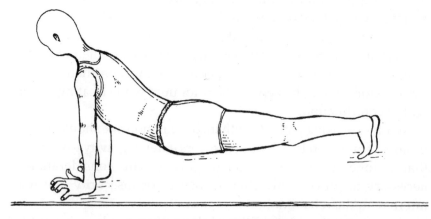

Fig. 3.2A: Prone on hand

rolling. Once the patient is able to efficiently go in to the sidelying position, he is taught asymmetrical push up with the upper limb and then trained to lower the legs from the bed onto the floor so that he can assume the position of sitting at the edge of the cot.

Sitting Balance

Once the patient achieves good head and trunk control, the therapist should progress to incorporate activities that will put demand on the patient's static and dynamic balance in sitting. The patient should be made to sit on a stable surface like cot or stool in a unsupported position and then the therapist gives perturbations (gentle pushes) in all directions. Alternately the patient may be asked to sit on unstable surface like a wobble board or vestibular ball without holding on to any support. Once the patient develops good static balance dynamic balance can be trained by giving swaying and rotational activities in sitting. Reaching out activities also improves the dynamic balance in sitting. The patient is made to sit on a vestibular ball then he is asked to hold a cane or medicine ball in his hand which is held in elevated position above the shoulder and then the patient may be made to do various movements of the trunk. Thus the exercises can be made more complicated for the patient.

Performing various functional tasks like dressing, grooming or feeding needs lot of repetition and goes a long way in making the patient functionally independent. The therapist should be skillful enough in allowing the patient to master a particular type of activity before progressing into the next realm of exercises.

Standing Activities

Once the patient has a good head and trunk control one needs to work on the control of the lower limb in order to make the patient stand successfully. Activities like unilateral bridging, crawling, kneeling and half kneeling helps in developing good pelvic and leg control. These exercises are progressed from supported position to unsupported position.

Sitting to standing can be practiced by making the patient sit on a chair or cot such that the feet are in proper contact with the ground. The patient is advised to lean slightly such that the center of gravity is brought between the feet, the therapist should stabilize the knee and support the pelvis thereafter the patient is encouraged to assume standing posture. Repetition of this task is essential till the patient masters the activity. The patient may be also taught standing by pulling on to the wall bar or parallel bar but for this the upper limb should be strong, nevertheless in the initial stages the support and assurance by the therapist is very important. Once the patient learns to stand, balance and weight transfer is taught. Posturography machine provides the important feedback to the patient which helps in improving the standing balance and control. Approximation given to the pelvis or to the shoulder also helps in facilitating stability in standing. In case the patient has tremor then ankle weights, a weighted belt or theraband can help in reducing them. Once the patient is stable in double support phase, weight transfer is practiced. Lastly in standing the patient is made to make a step with either limb in forward, backward and outward direction as a prerequisite to ambulation.

Gait Training

Gait training may be initially given in a parallel bar with foot marks. Footmarks are essential to reduce the tendency of the patient to walk with wide base of support. He needs constant verbal feedback regarding the step length, body rotation, accessory movements and trunk positions if the functional activity does not present itself as a whole procedural program. When the patient has to be progressed to walk outside a parallel bar, the therapist decides whether the patient needs to be given an assistive device, which is based upon the balance of the patient. Although walking aids do provide support to the patient, they also possess a problem because the patient will now need to control the position and movement of the device as well as themselves. Walker or cane may be used depending upon the patient's comfort.

Various coordination tests that were used as an assessment tool for incoordination are also used as exercises to improve coordination. The patient is asked to repeat each activity about 10 to 12 times during each session. The patient may be given these exercises as even home exercise program. At home patient can have multiple session with good rest in between them to avoid fatigue. Proximal fixation can be improved by using PNF techniques like rhythmic stabilization and approximation.

Frenkel's exercises are a very effective mean of improving the coordination. In fact it is very beneficial for patient with sensory ataxia. This coordination exercise which was first practiced by Dr HS Frenkel for treating cases of tabes dorsalis has been since then very widely used for all types of incoordination. This technique establishes control of movement by use of alternate sensory mechanism, which is intact, usually visual, sound and touch. The main principles of Frenkel's exercises are the following:

a. Concentration or attention
b. Precision
c. Repetition.

Technique

The patient is positioned in such a manner that he can see the movement. The therapist gives a concise explanation and even demonstrates the exercises so that the patient obtains a good mental picture of what he is expected to do. The patient should concentrate to perform a smooth and accurate movement. The speed of the movement is regulated by the therapist through the use of rhythmic counting, movement of her hand or the use of suitable music. The range of the movement is indicated by marking the spot (either number or alphabet) on which the foot or hand is to be placed. The exercises is repeated many times until the patient perfects it and is able to perform it with ease. The exercises are made more difficult by incorporating more movements and more joints into the exercise. Slower movements need more control than rapid movements hence alteration in the speed of consecutive movements is very essential to offer challenge to the patient.

Some Types of Frenkel's Exercises

Exercises for the Legs in Lying

- Flex and extend one leg by the heel sliding down a straight line on the table.
- Abduct and adduct hip smoothly with knee bent and heel on the table.
- Abduct and adduct leg with knee and hip extended by sliding the whole leg on the table.
- Flex and extend hip and knee with heel off the table.
- Flex and extend both the legs together with the heel sliding on the table.
- Flex one leg while extending the other.

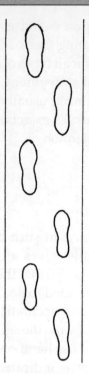

Fig. 3.2B: Foot marks to train gait in incoordination

- Flex and extend one leg while taking the other leg into abduction and adduction.

  Whether the patient slides the heels or lifts it off the bed he has to touch it to the marks indicated by the patient on the plinth. The patient may also be told to place the heel of one leg on various points of the opposite leg under the guidance of the therapist (Fig. 3.2 B).

Exercises for the Legs in Sitting

- One leg is stretched to slide the heel to a position indicated by a mark on the floor.
- The alternate leg is lifted to place the heel on the marked point.
- From stride sitting posture patient is asked to stand and then sit
- Rise and sit with knees together.

Exercises for the Legs in Standing

- In stride standing weight is transferred from one foot to other
- Place foot forward and backward on a straight line
- Walk along a winding strip

- Walk between two parallel lines
- Walk sideways by placing feet on the marked point
- Walk and turn around
- Walk and change direction to avoid obstacles.

Similar exercises can be devised for the upper limb wherein the patient may be directed to place the hand on the various points marked on the table or wall board to improve coordination of all the movements in the upper limb.

Certain diversional activities such as building with toy bricks or drawing on a black board, buttoning, combing, writing, typing are some of the activities that also improves the coordination.

SELF-ASSESSING QUESTIONS

Long and Short Essay

- Explain the role of cerebellum in motor function.
- What are the various causes of incoordination?
- Explain the clinical features of cerebellar lesion.
- Describe various tests to detect incoordination.
- Explain the management of cerebellar ataxia.
- Explain the management of sensory ataxia.
- What are the various PNF techniques that can be used to treat hypotonicity due to cerebellar conditions?
- Explain the principles and technique of Frenkel's exercises.
- Explain various exercises that can be given to improve proximal fixation in cerebellar lesion.
- Write a short note on Frederick's ataxia.

Short Answers

- What are various cerebellar connections?
- What is dysmetria?
- What is movement decomposition?
- What is the cause of hypotonicity in cerebellar lesion?
- What is Frederick's ataxia?
- Give two clinical featur of Frederick's ataxia.
- Define ataxia.
- Test for nystagmus.

4

Head Injury

Traumatic head injury is a condition in which an insult to the brain is caused to due any external force, which usually leads to alteration in the state of consciousness in the person that impairs the cognitive and physical function along with behavioral or emotional disturbances. These changes may be temporary or permanent and may cause partial or total disability.

In India the incidence of head injury has become very frequent due to lack of use of safety measures like helmets for two wheelers and seat belts for four wheelers. In addition the lack of application of traffic regulation adds on to the cause of increasing incidence. Most of the head injuries in our country are seen among younger age group with male having the upper hand.

MECHANISM OF INJURY

Traumatic brain injury is caused due to any external force and it could be associated with skull fracture in which case it is called as open head injury or it may happen in isolation without any skull fracture in which case it is called as closed head injury. The blow to head can cause brain injury at the site of impact and is called as coup injury or it may happen on the exactly opposite side of the brain and is called as contrecoup injury, e.g. When a patient falls on the forehead, the frontal part of the brain suffers damage due to direct impact of the brain (coup injury) but along with it there could be damage to the occipital part of the brain (contrecoup injury) that occurs due to bouncing back of the brain after its collision with the frontal bone that causes the occipital part to hit against the occipital portion of the skull.

Penetrating objects like bullets, missiles, sharp toys causes direct damage to the cells and vessels in the brain. Injury to the face and neck may also indirectly affect the brain by causing disturbance in the blood supply to the brain.

PATHOPHYSIOLOGY

The manifestation of brain damage could be due to primary damage or secondary damage.

Primary Damage

The brain can be primarily involved by acceleration force, deceleration force, rotational force or penetrating objects. These sources of injury can caused laceration, contusion, shearing, tension, or compression that causes primary damage to the brain structures. Primary damages are due to either a blow on the head by the object or head striking against the object. Areas in which the cranial vault is very irregular are more prone to get damage. Thus the anterior poles, undersurface of the temporal lobe, and undersurface of the frontal lobes are commonly injured.

Vascular lesion may also accompany due to either direct laceration of the blood vessels in the brain or due to lesion of the face, neck that can compromise the blood vessels supplying the brain. There can be direct injury to the nerve also, with optic, oculomotor, abducent, vestibulocochlear and facial being very sensitive.

Diffuse axonal injury or shearing injuries may be one of the most common ways of brain damage. Severe type of shear injury to the axon may even cause coma where as milder type of injury can cause spotty lesions leading to memory loss, decrease attention span, headaches, sleep disturbances and even seizures.

If penetrating object is of very high velocity like bullets then not only is the site of impact injured but even the surrounding areas due to the generation of shock waves as a result of high velocity. If the penetrating object is of low velocity like the toys then the insult is limited to only the site of impact.

Secondary Damage

This may results due to those causes that deprives the brain substances of proper blood supply which are the following:

Increased Intracranial Tensions

This occurs due to swelling or hematoma. Due to swelling there is distortion of the brain structures along with herniation of the brain structures to the opposite side. Increased intracranial tension have been associated with poor recovery and high mortality rates.

Cerebral Hypoxia or Ischemia

This occurs due to rupture or compression of the blood vessels in the brain. Hypoxia develops due to lack of blood supply to the brain or due to lack of adequate oxygen in the blood as a result of airway obstruction in associated chest injuries.

Intracranial Hemorrhage

This intensify the ischemic reaction by further causing lack of blood supply to those part of the brain supplied by the hemorrhaging blood vessels. Cell death following due to ischemia.

Electrolyte Imbalance and Acid Base Imbalance

Cell death occurs due to bursting of the swollen cells and also due to certain changes in the DNA within the cell.

Infection Secondary to Open Wounds

Infection of brain also leads to cell death.

Seizures due to Scarring or Pressure

Seizures is quite common following brain injury. It may occur immediately or after six months to two years following injury.

DEGREE OF SEVERITY OF HEAD INJURY

Although there are various factors that determines the amount of neurological deficit the patient may suffer following traumatic head injury but none is as better predictor as the severity of head injury. In fact one can say that the degree of severity of head injury is directly proportional to the amount of deficit that will follow. The severity of traumatic brain injury (TBI) is shown to directly correlate to the magnitude of the acceleration, deceleration and even the rotational forces.

Three basic category of head injury based upon the severity of brain damage have been identified which are as under

Mild Head Injury

These are those type of head injury in which there is minimal damage to the neuroanatomical structures with slight or no permanent impairment. This is a commonly encountered type of head injury. In fact repeated minor injuries over a time have been responsible for gradual loss of neurological or cognitive functions with marked cerebral atrophy. There appears to be primarily axonal disruption that is due to shear forces in the brainstem reticular formation and to some extent the cerebrum. The characteristic symptom of this type of injury consists of headache, dizziness, increased fatigability, decreased concentration power, poor memory and in some cases irritability. Diagnostic criteria for mild head injury consists of responses such as loss of consciousness for less than 20 minutes, Glasgow Coma Scale of more than 13, no focal neurological findings, no abnormality on CT scan and discharge from hospital within 48 hours.

Moderate Head Injury

These are those types who can be placed between mild and severe type of injury. The Glasgow Coma Scale ranges from anywhere between 8 to 13 and the post-traumatic amnesia lasting between 1 to 24 hours.

Severe Head Injury

These are those categories of head injury which is severe enough to produce an obvious disabling deficit but who regain the conscious activity status. Very few percentages of head injury patients do fall into this category.

Persistent vegetative state occurs in small percentage of head injury of patient because the injury is so severe that it doesn't allow restoration of consciousness. This condition occurs in acutely brain damaged patient after the stage of coma during which the patient is unaware of the surrounding environment, he can neither speak, and neither can communicate through any other means and does not exhibit any voluntary functions. However, certain activity like sleep-awake cycle, yawning, lip smacking, grimacing, withdrawal from painful stimuli, visual fixation and tracking presumably mediated through lower brain structures are usually preserved. This condition may persist for years.

CHANGES IN THE BODILY FUNCTIONS AFTER HEAD INJURY

Alteration is the State of Consciousness

The state of consciousness is usually altered in head injury patient due to depression of function of bilateral cerebral hemisphere, due to direct depression of brainstem function or due to destruction of brainstem activating system. Plum and Posner do not believe in direct relationship between the motor deficit to the depth of coma. According to them the parts of the brain which regulate the motor function and the part that regulate the state of alertness or consciousness are so distantly placed anatomically that it is quite impossible for them to be equated with respect of each other. The common state of consciousness, which the patient with head injury may be found to be in are as follows:

Coma

This is defined as complete arrest of all the cerebral function, a state of unresponsiveness to even strong noxious stimuli. The eyes are closed.

Stupor

This is also a state of generalized unresponsiveness but the patient reacts to painful stimuli through some bodily movements.

Obtundity:

This is a state of overt sleepiness and even on waking up the patient appears to be drowsy and disinterested in the surroundings.

Delirium

This is often noted when the patient comes out of the state of unconsciousness. Here the patient appears to be disoriented, fearful, will often misinterpret the sensory stimuli.

Clouding of Consciousness

This is a state of quite confusion, distractibility, faulty memory and slowed response to stimuli.

Sensorimotor

Motor abnormalities after head injury is common. The patient may have decerebrate rigidity or decorticate rigidity. Decerebrate represents extension attitude of all four limbs whereas decorticate manifests as flexion attitude in the upper limb and extension attitude of the lower limb. The condition may not be as well defined and over lap is inevitable.

Motor deficit could be in the form of hemiplegia, monoplegia with either presence of spasticity or flaccidity. One cannot set a fixed ideas regarding presentation of motor deficit in head injury cases, as there exist great variety. Either the patient may have extensor response in the lower limb with flexion response of the upper limb or *vice versa*. There could be a gradual progress from flaccidity to rigidity. Sometimes patient may have a generalized extensor response. The changes can be bilateral or unilateral. At times patient who was initially showing flexion response in the upper limb may suddenly show extension response which can be attributed to the physiological affect to the change in the amount of tissue compression. Daily changes in the tone may be noted which could be attributed to internal irritant or external factors. Involvement of the cerebellum or its pathway may cause impairment in timing, sequencing and coordination of voluntary movements. Dysarthria, or dysphasia may be seen. Some patient may also have dysphagia, visuospatial perceptual deficit. Sensation can be lost in various ways depending upon the site of injury. Most of the patients have balance disorder in the later stages, which can range from mild deviation to gross unsteadiness. Some of the patient may show presence of primitive reflexes.

Cranial nerve involvement is not unusual with certain cranial nerves like facial, optic, oculomotor, vestibulocochlear and abducent being commonly involved. The patient may have changes in the size, shape of pupil. The pupillary reaction to light may also show abnormalities. The movement of the eyeball may also be affected. The pharyngeal reflexes may be absent. Patient who have sustained severe head injury may even have a permanent physical deficit.

Cognitive, Emotional and Behavioral Changes

The abnormality in the memory and intellectual function of the patient may be temporary or permanent. Cognitive function of the patient may be affected due to generalized or focal lesion. Memory loss is very common after head injury. The patient may have posttraumatic amnesia, retrograde amnesia or anterograde amnesia. Retrograde amnesia is inability of the patient to recollect events that took place just before the injury. Posttraumatic amnesia is the time lapse between the injury till the time when the patient is supposed to have recovered back his memory function. Anterograde amnesia is inability of the patient to form new memory in future. This amnesia grossly retards the patient to learn new things and act as a serious handicap which severely restricts the rehabilitation outcome of the patient.

Many patient with head injury suffer trauma to the frontal lobe which is concerned with the control of executive function. Executive function regulates a person's behavior. According to Lezak four elements are there in executive function which are:

 i. Choosing a goal,
 ii. Developing a plan,
 iii. Execution of the plan,
 iv. Evaluation of the execution of the plan.

The patient has a reduced attention span, concentration ability, abstract reasoning, and decision making.

Emotional changes may be seen with lesion involving the orbitofrontal area of the brain. The patient may have euphoria, intolerance, irritability, inappropriate sexual behavior and unacceptable social or interpersonal behavior. The patient may have emotional lability of involuntary laughing or crying which will be irrespective of the emotions.

Behavioral changes may be like depression, impulsiveness or hyperactivity and these may be another stumbling block in the rehabilitation of the patient.

Clinical Rating System

The clinical rating system has been put forward in an attempt to put the various types of head injury patient into different categories based on their signs and symptoms. This rating system has simplified the description of patient due to its standardization. The commonly used rating scales are as follows:

Glasgow Coma Scale

This scale was first developed by Jennett B Teasdale and group based on visual, motor and verbal responses following TBI as below .

Eye opening E
   Spontaneous 4

To speech	3
To pain	2
Nil	1
Best motor response	M
Obeys command	6
Localizes response	5
Withdraws	4
Abnormal flexion	3
Extensor response	2
No response	1
Verbal response	V
Oriented	5
Confused conversation	4
Inappropriate words	3
Inappropriate sounds	2
No response	1

Coma score is E + M + V = 3 to 15

Rancho Los Amigos Level of Cognitive Function

This scale shows the sequence of cognitive and behavioral recovery that may be seen at different stages of head injury patient. The patient may become stagnant in his recovery at any stage. The information of this scale do help in guiding the evaluation and treatment protocol for TBI patients.

1. *No response:* Patient unresponsive to any stimuli.

2. *Generalized response:* The patient exhibit generalized mass unspecific response which is inconsistent and non-purposeful.

3. *Localized response:* The response is localized and specific to the stimulus but inconsistent.

4. *Confused agitated:* Usually very excited, shows agitated and non-purposeful behavior. Patient will be unable to recognize persons or object. Attention very brief and lack recalling ability.

5. *Confused inappropriate:* Response to simple command is fair, but cannot take complex command. Attention gross but easily distractible. Verbalization poor. Memory is also poor.

6. *Confused appropriate:* Response to simple command good. Behavior is goal directed but needs guidance. Attention span is improved. Shows carry over of learned activities to other tasks. Memory is better

but is still affected. Responses of the patient at times is wrong due to memory problems.

7. Automatic appropriate: Patient appears properly oriented, no confusion and is able to carry out all his routine activities but behaves more like a robot. Learning of new motor function is near normal. Initiate social and recreational interaction.

8. Purposeful appropriate: Patient is able to recall past and recent events with much ease. Does not need any supervision for learned activities. Able to carry over learned activities for applying in a new task. However patient has less tolerant to stress, abstract reasoning skills are affected and also judgement in emergency situation is not up to normal level.

Glasgow Outcome Scale

This scale also developed by Jennett's group is meant to categorize the clinical outcome of patients with TBI.

The five outcome categories are as follows:
1. *Death:* Self-evident criteria.
2. *Persistent vegetative state:* The patient is awake but not responsive to any form of stimuli.
3. *Severe disability:* The patient is conscious but is 24 hour dependent due to his cognitive, physical or behavioral disabilities. Even dysarthria and dysphasia is included.
4. *Moderated disability:* The patient is independent to carry-out his ADL activities in house as well as in the community although has disability. The patient may be having memory problem, personality changes, hemiparesis, dysphagia, ataxia, epilepsy or cranial nerve deficit.
5. *Good recovery:* Minor or no residual deficit. Patient can get back into normal social life and get back to job.

Rappaport Disability Rating Scale

This scale was developed by Rappaport and coworkers in an effort to desirable various degree of recovery after TBI. It ranges from 0 to 30 where 0 means no disability and 30 denotes death. The scale categorizes recovery in more detail manner and involves glass gow coma scale, assessment of cognitive ability, score with respect to the level of functional independency and even employability. The scale is as follows:

Total score	Level of disability
0	No disability
1	Mild disability
2 to 3	Partial
4 to 6	Moderate
7 to 11	Moderately severe
12 to 16	Severe
17 to 21	Extremely severe
22 to 24	Vegetative state
25 to 29	Extremely vegetative state
30	Death

ASSESSMENT

The evaluation of the head injury patient may not be always possible to be done as per a certain protocol of assessment due to the greater variety in the presentation of the patient and hence a flexible approach is necessary. Patients with head injury are frequently not cooperative during examination and even if they are cooperative most of the time they provide misleading information in their own assessment of the significant deficits present. Also it may not be possible to achieve a complete comprehensive assessment of the patient with TBI on a single visit.

The following may be used as a guidelines for evaluating head injury patients.

History: Information regarding the type of injury and its site is necessary. The duration of unconsciousness, present of lucid interval, external bleeding especially through the ears and nose needs to be found out. Some patient may also have leak of CSF through the nose. This information may not be obtained from the patient in acute stage and from those patient who are still in the state of confusion. Under these circumstances the history can be obtained from the patient or from the medical records.

The therapist should also find out about the educational status, previous job and home environment of the patient so as to canalize the rehabilitation process accordingly.

Client's and family data: This includes the patient's and family's goal, socioeconomic status of the patient, etc.

Past history: Whether the patient has had any previous head injury.

Observation: If the patient happens to be in the intensive care unit then one should note the setting of the various assistive and recording devices to which the patient is attached. For instance, it is necessary to see in which mode of ventilation the patient is or if he is on artificial ventilator. The various parameters on the pulse oximeter should be noted. Various tubing like catheters, etc. should be observed and noted.

Other observation includes that of attitude of various body parts of the patient, site and extent of scar, whether the scar appears to be healed or non-healed. The therapist should also look out for various signs of other associated injury or fracture. Presence of any swelling or oedema should also be noted.

Examination

Higher function: The consciousness of patient should be determined as per the Glasgow Coma Scale. The patient behavior is looked out for any signs of irritability, violence, or depression. Orientation should be checked. Speech and language, memory, intelligence, emotional response is also evaluated.

Only if the patient's consciousness is good and provided he is not confused then only it is possible to perform a complete evaluation of the patient. If the patient is not completely conscious then most of the examination consists of passive maneuvers. Those assessments which needs active cooperation of the patient may not be possible to be performed.

Cranial nerve testing: Certain nerves like the facial, abducent, vestibulocochlear and optic are very commonly involved and need to be assessed.

Sensory examination: All the sensations deep, superficial and cortical need to be assessed.

Reflexes: Deep and superficial reflexes.

Perceptual deficit: These should be evaluated in detail.

Motor: The motor dysfunction could be simple impairment or complex impairment and thus needs to be assessed separately.

Simple Impairments

Tone

Examination of tone begins by identifying muscle tension at rest. If the tension is increased it should be found whether the increase in tension is at muscle level (stiffness) or neurological level. Presence of increased tone in response to passive movement should be graded for which Modified Ashworth scale may be used.

0 – No increase in muscle tone.

1 – Slight increase in muscle tone manifested as catch and release at the end of the ROM during any movement.

1+ – Slightly more increased range manifested as a catch followed by release for at least half of the range.

2 – Increased resistance present throughout the range during passive movement but the part can be moved effortlessly.

3 – Considerable increase in muscle tone making passive movement difficult.

4 – Affected part remains in rigid flexion or extension.

Information obtained through EMG also indicates the excitability of the neuronal system. Brisk or exaggerated reflexes also identifies problem with the stretch reflex mechanism.

Muscle Flexibility or ROM

This is checked by doing passive range of motion assessment using a goniometer. The tightness of various muscles (especially biarticular muscles) need to be done.

Strength

The muscles become weak hence the power of the muscles need to be tested by doing manual muscle testing. However in those patients who have classical features of upper motor neuron, voluntary control testing is recommended.

Response or Reaction Time

It is measurement of time lapse between stimulus and response. It can be best tested by the use of EMG biofeedback or clinical EMG machines. The latency of the muscle activity denotes the reaction time. It can also be done in clinics based on observation using a stop watch but may cause technical errors.

Increase Moment Time

This is a direct indicator of the speed in which the movement is performed. Recording the time taken by patient to complete a given task provides an easy clinical tool. Video tape or movement analysis system can help to analyze function.

Endurance

Muscle endurance refers more to the ability of the muscle to produce the same level of contraction over time. It may be measured repeated muscle testing after giving set of activity to the muscle for a specific period of time. Detrimental studies used in EMG also shows fatigability of the muscles.

Complex Impairment

Basic Synergies

It is necessary to find if the patient has the basic synergy or pattern which is necessary to perform certain function in his activities of daily living. Are the basic higher level reflexes like equilibrium intact? Does the patient has good coordination?

Modification of the Basic Synergies

These functions are associated with the cerebellar function. This synergistic system helps to smoothen out the movement and provides adaptability. The patient is able to modify the basic synergies available to accomplish some unusual activity like catching the ball, walking on uneven surfaces, etc. Interlimb coordination should also be checked. Learning new activity is also dependent on this function.

Anticipatory Ability

Anticipatory reactions require combining past information with present information to make motor responses appropriate to internal and external needs. Examples of anticipatory functions includes contraction of gastrocnemius before forward reaching activities. Does the client step over objects or shape the hand for picking up the object. Almost all the motor functions has anticipatory component.

Use of Feedback

Use of feedback is very useful in head injury patient to relearn new skill. The client should be able to take the appropriate clue or hints given by the therapist to learn the skill. Does the patient possess the ability to correct his activity to meet the changing environmental condition.

Examination of Gait and Balance

They are very closely associated, in fact the walking activity requires three complex elements postural control, balance and extensor strength. The speed of walking, assistance needed and use of basic strategy at all joints during stance and swing phases should be assessed.

Autonomous nervous system function: The bowel, bladder and sweating function should be examined. The presence of marked trophic changes indicates autonomous dysfunction.

Functional disability status: All the basic functional activity should be checked for the level of independency. The Rappaport disability rating scale can be used as a guide.

MANAGEMENT

The management of the patient following head injury is generally determined by the state of the patient. Patient level of consciousness, alertness and ability to comprehend as well as learn taught skills are certain aspect on basis of which the treatment plan of the patient is designed. Patient in whom the active cooperation cannot be expected are the ones in whom the treatment consists of all passive maneuvers whereas patient with good contributory potential are usually trained through plenty of active maneuvers.

For practical purposes patient are classified into two category for treatment purposes as patient who are totally unconscious and patient who have regained their consciousness.

Management of Unconscious Patients

The treatment comprises of passive maneuvers that are necessary to maintain certain functions in the patient to prevent secondary problems later on. The treatment may be as follows:

Respiratory Care

The need for chest care is directly proportional to the extent of unconsciousness. The more number of days patient remains unconscious more intense and regular is the need for chest physiotherapy. Generally chest physiotherapy is given every 4 to 5 hourly. This is necessary to maintain good bronchial hygiene. Proper positioning of the patient associated with regular suctioning and nebulization enable the patient to have a relative clear lung. *Head low position should never be given to the head injury patient as it may cause a severe increase in the intracranial pressure that may prove to be hazardous.* Some patient may need ventilatory support that may increase the chances of lung infection due to intubation.

Preventing Contractures and Deformity

Passive movements should be given to the patient for all the joints including all the movements at that particular joint. Each movement may be repeated at least 8 to 12 times. Passive movements should be given every 3 to 4 hours and hence the therapist should guide the attender of the patient follow it up regularly.

Gentle rhythmic stretching is very essential especially for biarticular muscles as they become very prone to develop tightness. As the tone of the muscles increases the need for passive movement and stretching is even more to maintain range of motion at all joints. Use of appropriate splints and proper positioning is also desirable to prevent the chances of the patient developing any contracture.

Prevention and Treatment of Pressure Sores

Due to prolonged immobilization certain part of the body especially the ones with bony prominence are very prone to get subject to pressure sore due to lack of proper circulation to that area. Thus the lateral malleolus, lateral aspect of the knee, ischial tuberosity, sacrum, occiput are very likely to develop sore. The chances of sores can be kept to the minimum by taking certain preventive measures. The patient position should be changed from supine to side lying on either sides every 2 hourly at least. This will cause vascularization of almost all the areas of the body. The patient should be made to lie on water bed or air bed which helps in evenly distributing the weight throughout the body thus relieving some pressure from the above mentioned areas. The patient should be kept clean. The cloths should be regularly changed. Moisture increases the changes of skin infection and at the same time dry skin cause easy breakdown hence the patient's skin should be maintained in correct manner. Regular massage of pressure prone areas helps in increasing the circulation of these areas hence preventing pressure sores. Regular sponge bath helps in maintaining proper hygienic condition of the patients skin which offers resistance to development of unwanted infection. Presence of pressure sores retards the prognosis of the patient's condition by interfering with the rehabilitation process and should be discouraged from the first day.

In case the patient develops pressure sore then its healing can be accelerated by giving ozone therapy, UVR, IR or direct current. Ice massage given at the edges of the sores also helps in speeding the healing process. Sterile dressing should be applied following these physical therapy modalities.

Sensory Stimulation

Although the patient is unconscious effort should be made to stimulate the reticular activating system by using various sensory stimulation like auditory, tactile and proprioceptive stimulation (Figs 4.1A and B Plate 1).

Management of Conscious Patient

In patients who is conscious, active participation of the patient should be encouraged which in turn will speed up the rehabilitation process. The treatment may comprise of the following measures.

Improve Alertness or Arousal through Sensory Stimulation

The patient who is drowsy or confused need to be stimulated by make them more alert and awake. The therapist should encourage the patient's cooperation during the treatment. The main aim is to stimulate the reticular activating system by making the patient sit or even stand in the tilt table. The therapist should provide tactile, visual, auditory and proprioceptive stimulation to the patient that will send facilitatory signals to the brain and will enable the alert response to be provoked. Auditory stimulation can be given by speaking to the patient during the course of treatment. Introducing and casual addresses by the therapist are very important gestures that will have a beneficial effect.

Visual stimulation is given by showing familiar faces, objects or movement in the visual field of the patient.

Tactile stimulation is provided by the therapist's touch for carrying out various functional tasks. The touch of the patient also stimulates the receptors in the muscles and can be used for facilitating or inhibiting contraction of muscles.

Proprioceptive stimulation by giving traction and approximation at joint structures is very helpful in stimulating the arousal response in the patient.

Prevention of Spasticity

As hypertonicity generally sets in almost all head injury cases various measures need to be taken to keep them under control. Gentle passive movement, gradual rhythmic sustained stretch, prolonged icing for 20 minutes over the muscles, biofeedback, proper positioning are certain measures that needs to be employed for controlling spasticity.

Maximize the Patient's Functional Capacity

The main aim of this management is to improve the ROM, improve the control of voluntary movement, strengthening paretic muscles, improve the coordination, balance and teach various safety measures which will enable the patient to return back to the community.

The treatment should be wide spread over the period of time as the patient's attention span and endurance is very less.

Neuromuscular training can be given through the development sequence by inhibiting abnormal movement pattern and by facilitating normal movement pattern.

The patient may given activities like bridging, prone on elbow, on all fours, sidelying to sitting, sitting, kneeling, half kneeling, standing and walking.

Proper documentation is necessary of the entire event through-out the day. In fact the routine of the patient should be maintained in the register and the patient need to be reminded of various activities especially if the patient has memory problems. The patient may be given register with photo and names of various health professional visiting him so that each day's program can be entered. This will benefit both the patient and his acquaintance to know regarding the activities given to the patient.

Use of vestibular ball while training the patient for crawling, bridging, sitting balance helps in building the proprioceptive stimulation and teaches proper control to the patient.

Each task has various sub tasks which needs to be mastered by the patient so that he learns the actual activity using normal movement combination and performs it with precision. Like for training the patient to get up from bed, he may be taught to do asymmetrical push up with the trunk in partial rotation, then lower leg patterns are incorporated and finally the whole task of get up from side lying is practiced. *Repetition of activities* is key like any other neurological disorders. Ambulation training should always be done in upright position by training the patient in each and every phase of the gait cycle. If the patient's balance is poor then assistance may be used.

Functional electrical stimulation has been shown more effective than kinetic joint training in certain types of cases.

The upper extremity also appears to use specific synergies for hand use in different positions. Clients often can opens hand in out stretched arm position but will be unable to perform the same action when the elbow is flexed. Some patient with minimal functional deficit in the upper limb may be given some assistive devices or support for the hand so that they can perform some basic activity like eating, combing, writing, etc. This technique helps the shoulder and other proximal structures to produce appropriate movement sequences for hand use but does not facilitate hand function. The treatment however does provide whole task practice even though some basic component of the function is substituted by other means.

Reversing tasks in some patients helps in developing increased control by modifying a task or synergy as well as making the muscle work both eccentrically and concentrically. For instance lowering a glass of water on the table may help the patient in getting the glass close to the mouth by improving motor control of biceps during eccentric contraction.

Adding objects to the environment to expose the patient to various environment settings also helps in modifying the synergies and also develop adaptation strategies in the patient.

Development of High Level Skillful Functioning

These achievements may not be applicable to all head injury patients because not all head injury patients responds very favorably to rehabilitation measures. Patient belonging to the last two grades of cognitive grading may be considered as appropriate client for this training.

The safety awareness of the patient need to be improved because he is already in ambulatory stage. Balance and postural control training is very essential. Some patients may have good balance and postural control during normal walking but will have problems while trying to perform speedy actions. Dancing, basket ball, karate, tennis and certain other sports often promote additional progress in balance, sequencing, and speed of movement. The therapist should encourage those components of the activities that best address the deficits in the patient and plan out enjoyable activities that provide specific training for the deficits in balance, gait, upper extremity functions and so on (Figs 4.2A to D, Plate 2).

No matter at what level the patient is in teaching of functional skill is critical. The lowest level patient may learn to roll over, assisted eating or other basic ADL activities. Modern equipment can enhance all types of function. Computers communicate for those with severe dysarthria and power wheelchairs with switches to run lights, television are available. Advance technologies have gone yards infront in reducing handicap of the patient. One should remember that the main purpose of motion is for exploration that in turns puts the brains to its justified use. The therapist's uniqueness lies in the ability to do evaluation and effective intervention.

SELF-ASSESSING QUESTIONS

Long and Short Essay

- Classify head injuries and discuss the PT management of patient admitted in ICU following head injury.
- Describe PT management in acute stage of head injury.
- Describe management of head injury patient.
- Describe the physiotherapy management in detail in rehabilitation of head injury patient at various stages.
- Management of unconscious patient.
- PT management of head injury in conscious stage.
- Describe the various type of brain damages in head injury.
- Explain the various clinical rating scale for head injury patient.

Short Answers

- Signs of increased intracranial pressure.
- Different types of conscious state.
- Scale for cognitive dysfunction.
- What is diffuse axonal injury?
- What is countre coup injury?

5

Parkinsonism

Parkinsonism or Parkinsonian syndrome group is of disorders which manifests as tremor, disturbances in voluntary movement (rigidity, bradykinesia or akinesia) and impairment in the balance and automatic reactions.

This syndrome do occur in various conditions, of which Parkinson's disease is quite common.

Parkinson's disease was observed by James Parkinson in the year 1817. It took about 100 years to be well verse with the pathology of this disease condition and the treatment was partially achieved by the introduction of Levo-dopa in the year 1960.

ETIOLOGY

a. *Idiopathic:* The etiology is not understood. Example of this type of parkinsonism is Parkinson's disease, where there is degeneration of neurons in the substantia nigra and corpus striatum (Striatonigral pathway). It occurs usually in late adult life, progress slowly, and kills the patient by 10-15 years after the onset.

b. *Vascular:* Multi-infarct disease (atherosclerotic parkinsonism).

c. *Infection:* Infection by various viruses, most commonly influenza virus may be causing parkinsonism like features. It is termed as encephalitis lethargica that causes focal insult to the brain matter.

d. *Due to toxicity:* Certain toxic chemicals like manganese, carbon disulfide, carbon monoxide, cyanide exposed in various occupation can cause diffuse damage to the brain exhibiting parkinsonian syndromes.

e. *Various drugs:* Phenothiazines, butyrophenones, tetrabenazine can cause Parkinsonism.

f. Multiple system degeneration that occurs in conditions like Alzheimer disease shy-Drager syndrome, supranuclear ophthalmoplegia, Wilson s disease, etc. can cause parkinsonism.

g *Metabolic:* Abnormal calcium metabolism can cause disposition of calcium in the basal ganglia causing parkinsonism.

h *Traumatic:* Multiple brain damage commonly encountered in boxers usually causes parkinsonism. This types of parkinsonism are called as punch boxers syndrome.

PATHOLOGY

Due to degeneration of neurons in the striatonigral pathway, there is deficiency in the level of dopamine. Dopamine is a neurotransmitter in the striatonigral pathway that inhibits the excitation of the cholinergic pathway, which has acetylcholine as the neuro-

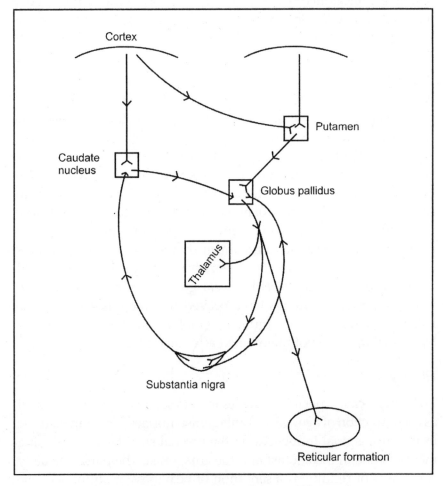

Fig. 5.1: Striatonigral pathway from caudate nucleus and putamen to substantia nigra and back

transmitter. Thus decrease in the dopamine level, removes the inhibitory influence on the cholinergic pathway causing excessive excitation of the extrapyramidal system (reticulo and rubro), which causes increased tone in the agonist and antagonist. This gives rise to rigidity and bradykinesia (Fig. 5.1).

The exact cause of tremors is not properly known.

CLINICAL FEATURES

Disturbances in the Voluntary Movement

Although there is no involvement of corticospinal tract but still the patient exhibit difficulty in the performance of voluntary movement which is mainly due to two abnormal features seen in parkinsonism which are as follows:

Bradykinesia

According to Jacksonian's principle, this is a negative feature of parkinsonism. It means slowing of movement with decrease in the amplitude and intensity of contraction. There is plenty of time lag between patients desire to act and the actual action produced. This is called as increased reaction time. There is also an increase in the movement time, which is the total time needed by the patient to complete a single sequence of movement. These disabilities are more pronounced while performing precision function involving distal parts of body. The exact mechanism that leads to bradykinesia is not known, but however, it is theoretically presumed that it could be because of difficulty of the basal ganglia to integrate sensory information. EMG studies have proved that there is a lot of time lapse before the actual recruitment of motor units and also the firing by motor units are not maintained after its initiation.

Rigidity

This can be called positive features in parkinsonism. It is manifested as cocontraction of agonist and antagonist muscles due to an increase in the supraspinal influences on the normal spinal system causing increase tone in the agonist and the antagonist. The patient usually complains of rigidity as a sensation of heaviness or stiffness of the limbs.

Rigidity may involve all the body parts and may be symmetrically or asymmetrically distributed. It occurs in three forms:

Lead pipe: In this the resistance is constant and uniform.

Cogwheel: In this the resistance is intermittent but uniform.

Akinesia: It is an inability to initiate movement. It occurs due to severe rigidity.

Postural Disturbances

The patient's ability to maintain both static and dynamic posture or balance is severely impaired due to combined influence of disturbance in vestibular, proprioception, visual, and righting reactions. Also there is loss of protective reaction of upper limb extension during a fall causing a fear of injury to the patient.

Tremors

This is defined as involuntary oscillations of body parts at frequency ranging from 3.5 to 7 Hz. It is one of the cardinal signs of parkinsonism and in many patients this is the first sign of disease. The tremors occur due to uninhibited activity of the basal ganglia-cortico-thalamus circuit as a result of degeneration of the striato-nigral pathway. The tremors seen in parkinsonism is resting tremors which is absent in sleep and increase with voluntary efforts or even emotional excitement. The tremor is typically the pin-rolling type observed in finger, tremors may also be occasionally seen in the lips and tongue.

Gait

Combination of movement and sequential movement task are grossly affected in parkinsonism. Thus parkinsonism patient exhibits severe difficulty in walking.

Initially, there is only lack of associated movements (like swinging of arm while walking). Later on the gait becomes slow, shuffling gait with small steps. The initiation of walking is difficult, but after initiation the patient may walk fast with small steps in a bend attitude and eventually run as if to catch up with his center of gravity. This is called *Festinating gait*. On the other hand, patient may also have freezing of gait. In this case, patient walks quite well initially with relatively larger steps but eventually shuffles at the same place without proceeding further. This is called as *Freezing*. Some patient may have difficulty in stopping suddenly and needs some external force to bring their gait to stop.

Facial Attitude

Parkinsonism patient suffer from masked or expressionless face. The person appears to be continuously staring. There is constant frowning in majority of individuals. The skin appears shiny and greasy with increased salivation and drooling due to autonomic dysfunction.

Posture

Stooped attitude with flexed trunk and the limbs (Figs 5.2A and 5.2B Plate 3, 5.3A and 5.3B Plate 3).

Speech

Parkinsonism patient have slurred speech. Hand writing is micrographia (the size of the letter gradually becomes smaller and smaller).

Dysphagia

It may be seen in half percent of parkinsonian patients.

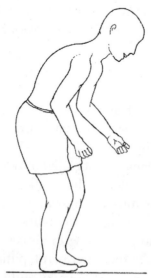

Fig. 5.2A: Posture lateral view (in parkinsonism)

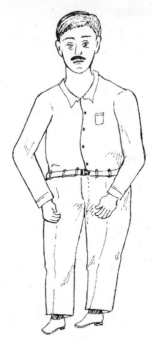

Fig. 5.3A: Anteroposterior view (in parkinsonism)

Visual Difficulties

Blurring of vision, decreased blinking that causes eye strain and rarely diplopia. Glabellar tap reflex fails to habituate. Oculogyric crisis may occur sometimes.

Asthenia

Generalized weakness may be seen, although, these are not due to direct involvement of lower motor neuron but mainly due to deconditioning and rigidity.

Reflexes

Deep tendon reflexes are not directly affected, but however, they may be difficult to elicit or may be reduced in amplitude due to rigidity. Plantar response is down going.

Sensory Involvement

Inactivity and stiffness may cause generalized body pain in 50 percent of cases along with cramps and tight muscles.

Psychological Impairment

Dementia is very common in about 40 percent of parkinsonism patients. Depression, lack of motivation, over-dependency are other psychological manifestations noted in parkinsonism patients.

Perceptual deficits like difficulty in vertical perception, body scheme, body image disorder and topographical disorientation have been noted.

Secondary Complications

1. Decrease in joint range and flexibility causing tightness and contracture. Contractures are seen in hip and knee flexors, hip adductors, trunk flexors, neck flexors, shoulder adductors, elbow flexors, wrist and finger flexors. Kyphotic deformity is common due to the patient's abnormal attitude.
2. Muscle atrophy and weakness are secondary dysfunction.
3. Cardiopulmonary changes: Deconditioning of the cardiovascular and respiratory system is common due to decreased activity and kyphotic posture that causes compression of the vital structure in the thorax.
4. Osteoporosis: Prolonged inactivity and poor diet intake causes osteoporosis. Moreover, frequent fall always increase the likelihood of a fracture.
5. Edema: May occur in the distal parts of the foot due to venous pooling as a result of decreased pumping action of calf muscles.
6. Skin infections like dermatitis can occur due to increased secretion by sweat and sebaceous glands.

ASSESSMENT

The assessment given below is from physiotherapy point of view:

For convenience and practical purpose the assessment of parkinsonism patient is divided into various parts which are as follows:

Observations

The overall behavior of the patient should be noted. The posture of the patient should be observed in lying, supine and in standing with emphasize on the attitude of the different parts. The patient facial attitude should also be noted. The skin condition, presence of any superficial lesions, should be described. The type of tremors should be noticed with its variation to different activity and situation. The presence of any disuse wasting of the muscles should also be observed.

Examination

Higher functions like memory, intelligence, speech, orientation, and behavior should be checked.

Motor Examination

Tone

This should be checked by slow passive movement unlike spasticity, which is checked by fast jerky passive movement. It is necessary to find out the distribution and extent of hypertonicity. In parkinsonism the hypertonicity is rigidity which is either lead pipe or cogwheel.

Tightness

Testing of all biarticular muscles of the upper limb and the lower limb for tightness is necessary.

ROM

The range of motion of all the joints of the upper limb and the lower limb should be assessed with a goniometer. Spinal mobility can be checked by use of tape. Usually, as the patient has a predominantly flexed posture the extension ranges are reduced.

MMT

Although the muscle power is not directly involved, the deconditioning effect of immobilization causes a generalized weakness, which should be assessed by Manual muscle test. Due to the presence of bradykinesia and rigidity the performance of isotonic contraction of the muscle is affected hence the muscle testing is best done using isometric contraction of the muscle by the procedure of Test position in MMT, e.g. for checking the abductors of the shoulder the persons arm is passively taken to 90 degree of abduction and then he is asked to hold while the therapist tries to break the patient's hold.

Test for Bradykinesia

It has been found that it is bradykinesia which has a negative influence on the patient's functional recovery unlike earlier belief which considered rigidity to be the main factor interfering with the patients recovery. Testing of bradykinesia is done by timing the various activity undertaken by the patient. However, the activity selected should be the one that forms the normal pattern, which will be beneficial for the patient in learning his ADL activities, e.g. Examples, for the upper limb the patient may be asked to take the hand to the mouth or touch the opposite shoulder or touch the head. The time taken by the patient to complete this task immediately after the instruction is given is noted. This will include even the reaction time (time taken by the patient to initiate the action after the instruction is made). More complex and skillful activity should also be tested which includes dressing activity or tying the shoe lace, etc.

For the trunk, bending activities, rotation and lateral bending should be timed.

For the lower limb, flexion adduction pattern or flexion abduction pattern may be selected to find the extent of bradykinesia. In standing bradykinesia for the lower limb can be tested by asking the patient to put a step forward and then take it back. The same may be repeated by the other leg.

Tapping the foot on the ground and then counting the number of tapping for a minute is another way of checking for bradykinesia that involves repeated alternating movement.

Sensory Examination

The sensations are not directly involved but the patient may have altered sensation, which should be assessed as they may interfere in rehabilitation.

Reflexes

The superficial and deep reflexes are checked. They may be normal or difficult to elicit due to the presence of rigidity. The plantars are down going and the abdominal reflexes may be difficult to elicit as a result of trunk rigidity.

Coordination Assessment

Coordination assessment can be done by various tests like finger-nose-finger test, alternate supination and pronation, heel-shin test, Tandem walking, etc.

Balance

The patient's balance should be checked in different postures viz., sidelying, sitting and standing. Static balance can be checked by giving perturbations (gentle, sudden pushes in all directions). Static balance should be checked in sitting and standing. Dynamic balance should by checked by asking the patient to perform various activities of the trunk and limbs like trunk rotation, lateral bending, reaching out, picking out and finding the patient's stability while he performs these activities.

Gait Assessment

The gait assessment should include whether the patient is walking independently or with assistance. The type of gait, i.e. whether he has freezing or festinating should be observed. Various gait parameters like step length, stride length, step width, cadence should be measured.

Chest Assessment

As a result of reduced activity and stooped posture, the patient with parkinsonism is prone to have some respiratory deconditioning, hence, the following chest assessment should be carried out:
- Finding out the breathing pattern.
- Measuring the inspiratory to expiratory ratio.
- Measuring the chest expansion at three levels, viz, at the level of anterior axillary fold, level of nipple, and two inches above the umbilicus.

Functional Evaluation

All the activities of the daily living namely eating, combing, washing, dressing, reaching out activities should be checked for the level of independency and also the speed at which it is done. The Yoehn and Yahr staging of Parkinsonism as well as Unified Parkinsonism Rating Scale can be used to know the severity of the disease. These are as follows:

HOEHN AND YAHR STAGING OF PARKINSON'S DISEASE

1. Stage One
    i. Signs and symptoms on one side only.
    ii. Symptoms mild.
    iii. Symptoms inconvenient but not disabling.
    iv. Usually presents with tremor of one limb.
    v. Friends have noticed changes in posture, locomotion and facial expression.

2. Stage Two
   i. Symptoms are bilateral.
   ii. Minimal disability.
   ii. Posture and gait affected.

3. Stage Three
   i. Significant slowing of body movements.
   ii. Early impairment of equilibrium on walking or standing.
   iii. Generalized dysfunction that is moderately severe.

4. Stage Four
   i. Severe symptoms.
   ii. Can still walk to a limited extent.
   iii. Rigidity and bradykinesia.
   iv. No longer able to live alone.
   v. Tremor may be less than earlier stages.

5. Stage Five
   i. Cachectic stage.
   ii. Invalidism complete.
   iii. Cannot stand or walk.
   iv. Requires constant nursing care.

This rating system has been largely supplanted by the Unified Parkinson's Disease Rating Scale, which is much more complicated.

UNIFIED PARKINSON DISEASE RATING SCALE (UPDRS)

The UPDRS is a rating tool to follow the longitudinal course of Parkinson's Disease. It is made up of the 1) mentation, behavior, and mood, 2) ADL, and 3) motor sections. These are evaluated by interview. Some sections require multiple grades assigned to each extremity. A total of 199 points are possible. 199 represents the worst (total disability), 0—no disability.

I. MENTATION, BEHAVIOR, MOOD

Intellectual Impairment

0. One
1. Mild (consistent forgetfulness with partial recollection of events with no other difficulties)
2. Moderate memory loss with disorientation and moderate difficulty handling complex problems

3. Severe memory loss with disorientation to time and often place, severe impairment with problems
4. Severe memory loss with orientation only to person, unable to make judgments or solve problems

Thought Disorder

0. None
1. Vivid dreaming
2. "Benign" hallucination with insight retained
3. Occasional to frequent hallucination or delusions without insight, could interfere with daily activities
4. Persistent hallucination, delusions, or florid psychosis.

Depression

0. Not present
1. Periods of sadness or guilt greater than normal, never sustained for more than a few days or a week
2. Sustained depression for >1 week
3. Vegetative symptoms (insomnia, anorexia, abulia, weight loss)
4. Vegetative symptoms with suicidality

Motivation Initiative

0. Normal
1. Less of assertive, more passive
2. Loss of initiative or disinterest in elective activities
3. Loss of initiative or disinterest in day to say (routine) activities
4. Withdrawn, complete loss of motivation

II. ACTIVITIES OF DAILY LIVING

Speech

0. Normal
1. Mildly affected, no difficulty being understood
2. Moderately affected, may be asked to repeat
3. Severely affected, frequently asked to repeat
4. Unintelligible most of time

Salivation

0. Normal
1. Slight but noticeable increase, may have nighttime drooling
2. Moderately excessive saliva, hay minimal drooling

3. Marked drooling

Swallowing

0. Normal
1. Rare choking
2. Occasional choking
3. Requires soft food
4. Requires NG tube or G-tube

Handwriting

0. Normal
1. Slightly small or slow
2. All words small but legible
3. Severely affected, not all words legible
4. Majority illegible

Cutting Food/Handing Utensils

0. Normal
1. Somewhat slow and clumsy but no help needed
2. Can cut most foods, some help needed
3. Food must be cut, but can feed self
4. Needs to be fed

Dressing

0. Normal
1. Somewhat slow, no help needed
2. Occasional help with buttons or arms in sleeves
3. Considerable help required but can do something alone
4. Helpless

Hygiene

0. Normal
1. Somewhat slow but no help needed
2. Needs help with shower or bath or very slow in hygienic care
3. Requires assistance for washing, brushing teeth, going to bathroom
4. Helpless

Turning in Bed/ Adjusting Bed Clothes

0. Normal
1. Somewhat slow no help needed
2. Can turn alone or adjust sheets but with great difficulty
3. San initiate but not turn or adjust alone
4. Helpless

Falling Unrelated to Freezing

0. None
1. Rare falls
2. Occasional, less than one per day
3. Average of once per day
4. >1 per day

Freezing When Walking

0. Normal
1. Rare, may have start hesitation
2. Occasional falls from freezing
3. Frequent freezing, occasional falls
4. Frequent falls from freezing

Walking

0. Normal
1. Mild difficulty, day drag legs or decrease arm swing
2. Moderate difficultly requires no assist
3. Severe disturbance requires assistance
4. Cannot walk at all even with assist

Tremor

0. Absent
1. Slight and infrequent, not bothersome to patient
2. Moderate, bothersome to patient
3. Severe, interfere with many activities
4. Marked, interferes with many activities

Sensory Complaints Related to Parkinsonism

0. None
1. Occasionally has numbness, tingling, and mild aching

2. Frequent, but not distressing
3. Frequent painful sensation
4. Excruciating pain

III. MOTOR EXAM

Speech

0. Normal
1. Slight loss of expression, diction,volume
2. Monotone, slurred but understandable, mod. impaired
3. Marked impairment, difficult to understand
4. Unintelligible

Facial Expression

0. Normal
1. Slight hypomymia, could be poker face
2. Slight but definite abnormal diminution in expression
3. Mod. hypomimia, lips parted some of time
4. Masked or fixed face, lips parted 1/4 of inch or more with complete loss of expression

Tremor at Rest

Face

0. Absent
1. Slight and infrequent
2. Mild and present most of time
3. Moderate and present most of time
4. Marked and present most of time

Right Upper Extremity (RUE)

0. Absent
1. Slight and infrequent
2. Mild and present most of time
3. Moderate and present most of time
4. Marked and present most of time

Left upper extremity (LUE)

0. Absent
1. Slight and infrequent

2. Mild and present most of time
3. Moderate and present most of time
4. Marked and present most of time

Right lower extremity (RLE)

0. Absent
1. Slight and infrequent
2. Mild and present most of time
3. Moderate and present most of time
4. Marked and present most of time

Left lower extremity (LLE)

0. Absent
1. Slight and infrequent
2. Mild and present most of time
3. Moderate and present most of time
4. Marked and present most of time

Action or Postural Tremor

Right Upper Extremity

0. Absent
1. Slight, present with action
2. Moderate, present with action
3. Moderate present with action and posture holding
4. Marked, interferes with feeding

Left upper extremity

0. Absent
1. Slight, present with action
2. Moderate, present with action
3. Moderate present with action and posture holding
4. Marked, interferes with feeding

Rigidity

Neck

0. Absent
1. Slight or only with activation

2. Mild/moderate
3. Marked, full range of motion
4. Severe

Right upper extremity

0. Absent
1. Slight or only with activation
2. Mild/moderate
3. Marked, full range of motion
4. Severe

Left upper extremity

0. Absent
1. Slight or only with activation
2. Mild/moderate
3. Marked, full range of motion
4. Severe

Right lower extremity

0. Absent
1. Slight or only with activation
2. Mild/moderate
3. Marked, full range of motion
4. Severe

Left lower extremity

0. Absent
1. Slight or only with activation
2. Mild/moderate
3. Marked, full range of motion
4. Severe

Finger taps

Right

0. Normal
1. Mild slowing, and/or reduction in amp.
2. Moderate impaired. Definite and early fatiguing, may have occasional arrests

3. Severely impaired. Frequent hesitations and arrests.
4. Can barely perform

Left

0. Normal
1. Mild slowing, and/or reduction in amp.
2. Moderate impaired. Definite and early fatiguing, may have occasional arrests
3. Severely impaired. Frequent hesitations and arrests.
4. Can barely perform

Hand Movements (Open and Close Hands in Rapid Succession)

Right

0. Normal
1. Mild slowing, and/or reduction in amp.
2. Moderate impaired. Definite and early fatiguing, may have occasional arrests
3. Severely impaired. Frequent hesitations and arrests.
4. Can barely perform

Left

0. Normal
1. Mild slowing, and/or reduction in amp.
2. Moderate impaired. Definite and early fatiguing, may have occasional arrests
3. Severely impaired. Frequent hesitations and arrests.
4. Can barely perform

Rapid Alternating Movements (Pronate and Supinate Hands)

Right

0. Normal
1. Mild slowing, and/or reduction in amp.
2. Moderate impaired. Definite and early fatiguing, may have occasional arrests
3. Severely impaired. Frequent hesitations and arrests.
4. Can barely perform

Left

0. Normal
1. Mild slowing, and/or reduction in amp.
2. Moderate impaired. Definite and early fatiguing, may have occasional arrests
3. Severely impaired. Frequent hesitations and arrests.
4. Can barely perform

Leg Agility (Tap Heel on Ground, Amp should be 3 Inches)

Right

0. Normal
1. Mild slowing, and/or reduction in amp.
2. Moderate impaired. Definite and early fatiguing, may have occasional arrests
3. Severely impaired. Frequent hesitations and arrests.
4. Can barely perform

Left

0. Normal
1. Mild slowing, and/or reduction in amp.
2. Moderate impaired. Definite and early fatiguing, may have occasional arrests
3. Severely impaired. Frequent hesitations and arrests.
4. Can barely perform

Arising from Chair (Pt. Arises with Armsfolded Across Chest)

0. Normal-slow, may need more than one attempt
2. Pushes self up from arms or seat
3. Tends to fall back, may need multiple tries but can arise without assistance
4. Unable to arise without help

Posture

0. Normal erect
1. Slightly stooped, could be normal for older person
2. Definitely abnormal, mod. stooped, may lean to one side

3. Severely stooped with kyphosis
4. Marked flexion with extreme abnormality of posture

Gait

0. Normal
1. Walks slowly, may shuffle with short steps, no festination or propulsion
2. Walks with difficulty, little or no assistance, some festination, short steps or propulsion
3. Severe disturbance, frequent assistance
4. Cannot walk

Postural Stability (Retropulsion Test)

0. Normal
1. Recovers unaided
2. Would fall if not caught
3. Falls spontaneously
4. Unable to stand

Body Bradykinesia/ Hypokinesia

0. None
1. Minimal slowness, could be normal, deliberate character
2. Mild slowness and poverty of movement, definitely abnormal, or dec. amp. of movement
3. Moderate slowness, poverty, or small amplitude
4. Marked slowness, poverty, or amplitude

INVESTIGATION

EMG may done to find out the level of rigidity and also to know the increase in the reaction time and movement time. Pulmonary function test can done to check the patient vital capacity.

MANAGEMENT

Unlike earlier days, today the role of a physiotherapist in managing a Parkinson's disease patient starts in the acute stages itself, mainly to maintain the musculoskeletal flexibility (with equal emphasize on the thoracic expansion) and to advice the patient to lead an active livestyle. This is essential to minimize deconditioning and to prevent psychological decline.

The physiotherapy treatment methods should be directed towards achieving the main goal that is improving the functional performance in everyday life.

In order to achieve this long-term goal various short-term goal has to be first achieved:

1. Maintaining or improving the ROM at all joints.
2. Preventing any contracture or deformity especially of the upper limb and trunk.
3. Prevent any deconditioning of the muscles or cardiorespiratory system.
4. Encourage the patient to lead an active lifestyle.
5. Improve the physical fitness of the patient.
6. Prevent the influence of psychosocial factors like depression and over dependency on the patient.

However, the goals and priority of the treatment may be different from patient to patient and that depends upon the severity of the clinical signs, the patient's needs, and also his motivation. The major roles for the physiotherapist is to see that the patient leads an active life with near normal independency, to gain musculs skeletal flexibility, and a good physical fitness.

The following measures may be used as a guideline for treating patient with parkinsonism but there are no fixed methods of treating parkinsonism which demands lot of study and work in this condition.

REDUCTION OF RIGIDITY

Rigidity has been found to reduce, to some extent, by generalized relaxation technique. Generalized relaxation can be obtained by vestibular stimulation that can be achieved by various rocking techniques. Rocking can be achieved by the use of adult vestibular ball, rocking or rotating chair, and cradle. Rhythmic initiation, which is a technique of PNF, can be used to reduce rigidity. This technique, which involves progression of exercise from passive to active assisted to active without any increase in tone, has been found to be very effective in reducing rigidity of the trunk.

Generalized relaxation techniques like Jacobsons technique of progressive relaxation, yogasana, transdental meditation, biofeedback, savasana, etc. can also be used.

MAINTAINING THE FLEXIBILITY
OF MUSCULOSKELETAL SYSTEM

Flexibility of the musculoskeletal systems can be maintained by encouraging the patient to lead an active life. However, passive exercise by the therapist or the relatives may be of help in maintaining or increasing flexibility. Passive exercise to the patient should be given at least 2 to 3 times in a day. As the patient has a predominantly flexed posture the mobility exercises should involve plenty of extension activity. Passive stretching should be given for all shortened muscles. Some times braces may be used for prolonged stretching of tight muscles. PNF technique of hold relax or contract relax can be used to bring about lengthening of contracted muscles and thus increase the ROM of various joint. PNF pattern of flexion abduction with elbow extension for the upper limb, extension abduction with knee extension for the lower limb and neck extension with rotation to either side should be emphasized to overcome the flexed posture of a parkinsonism patient. During the extension movement the patient should be asked breath in. This will help in increasing the thoracic expansion of the patient.

Apart from passive exercise, the patient should be encouraged to maintain joint mobility through active exercises and auto-stretching. Calisthenics exercises in supine, sitting or standing posture is of great use to patients of parkinsonism. As there is an tendency in parkinsonism patients to develop overall flexed posture, this may be countered by various simple stretching programs like standing erect with arms in elevation (over the head) against a wall or corner of the room, and the patient should try and stretch out his whole body. Also, the patient should be instructed to lie supine with a pillow under the upper thorax, which can play a significant role in stretching the upper limb and upper thoracic spine (Figs 5.4A and B).

BALANCING TRAINING

The balancing training should always be begun from a low center of gravity level to higher center of gravity level. In sitting at the edge to the cot, the patient may be given perturbation to develop his static stability. Dynamic stability in sitting may be developed by weight shift, shifting from one end of the cot the other, and by incorporating various reaching out activities. Trunk rotation

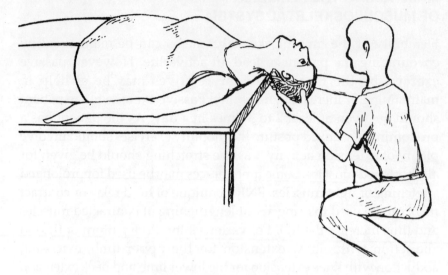

Fig. 5.4A: Neck extension PNF pattern in parkinsonism

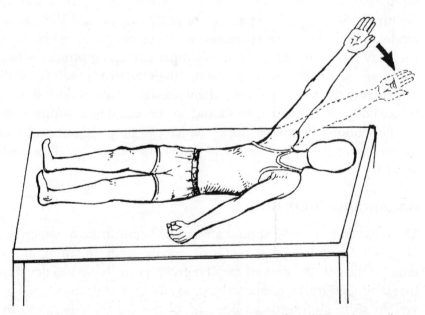

Fig. 5.4B: Flexion abduction upper limb PNF pattern for parkinsonism patient

activities both in horizontal plane and in diagonal manner should be trained in the patient. Sitting activities on an adult vestibular ball has also been found to be very effective in training the patient's balance. Once the patient is quite stable in sitting the therapist can progress to train him to achieve standing balance. In standing, the patient may be trained for weight shift from one limb to other, trunk rotation, and other bending and reaching out activities. (Fig. 5.5, Plate 3)

One should always remember that training should be done in different sensory and environmental conditions and preferably in his house. The patient's anticipatory and automatic response should be trained.

COORDINATION EXERCISES

The various tests that are used for testing coordination both in the upper limb and lower limb can be used as exercises for training coordination. Frenkel's exercises can also be used.

BREATHING OR THORACIC EXPANSION EXERCISES

Diaphragmatic and segmental breathing exercises should be taught to improve the patient's vital capacity. Exercises like balloon blowing or incentive spirometry gives the patient visual feedback and is quite effective in improving the thoracic expansion.

FUNCTIONAL REEDUCATION OR TRAINING

Functional reeducation in parkinsonism means task and context related practice. Working on the musculoskeletal complication without any training in the functional task is not going to suffice in the training of the parkinsonism patient. Sufficient evidence proves that visual cues and auditory cues stimulates learning of the functional task quicker and also overcomes the slowness in performance to some extent.

Auditory cues like clap, musical beat, metronomes, etc. have been used very effectively in improving the performance of activities of daily living especially gait.

Improvement in the functional task by overcoming bradykinesia has been found through training that involves repetition of that function several times in a day over a period of 2-3 months. It is essential that the therapist give certain basic biomechanical explanations or tips which help the patient in overcoming the difficulty by many folds.

The patient should be trained for various activities like turning in the bed, lying to sitting, sitting to standing, walking straight, and walking around a chair or cot. Turning around and sudden stopping imposes severe difficulty to a parkinsonism patient. This has to be trained once the patient masters the other challenges in walking.

Gait can be very well trained by use of visual cues in the form of foot markers on the floor. In comparison to blocks or sticks that were conventionally used to overcome freezing, parallel lines drawn in front of the patient has been found to be quite effective for the same. The patient learns to step over the lines quite comfortably as compared to wooden blocks. *Use of a walker or parallel bar is not advisable in treatment of parkinsonism because the confined nature of this gait training apparatus only increases the freezing.* Once the patient is able to walk in the empty room quite comfortably then he should be trained to walk in the environment of the house. It is essential to keep track of the time taken by the patient to cover a particular distance and the speed of walking so that it could be compared later on to see the extent of improvement.

Similarly other precision activities of daily living like eating, dressing, washing, etc. should be trained by overcoming the bradykinesia.

IMPROVING THE PHYSICAL FITNESS

Cardiovascular and respiratory conditioning can be achieved by involving the patient in various aerobics exercises like calisthenics, static cycling, swimming, etc. It has been shown that the parkinsonism individual who performed regular aerobic exercises produced higher percentage predicted maximum O_2 consumption values than those who were sedentary.

However, this conditioning program is possible only in mild to moderate types of parkinsonism patient. The author doesn't feel its possible to train patient with severe parkinsonism.

IMPROVEMENT IN THE PSYCHOLOGICAL WELL-BEING

Once the patient learns to lead a relatively active functional life he will feel much more confident and independent that it will reduce the depression or over dependency of the patient.

One should note that it is not fair to give false assurance to a parkinsonism patient regarding his improvement because total recovery is not possible. The best that could be done through physiotherapy is maximizing the patient's functional independency.

SELF-ASSESSING QUESTIONS

- Draw diagram of striatonigral pathway and give the clinical feature of parkinsonism.
- What are the clinical features and management of parkinsonism?
- Difference between spasticity and rigidity.
- Describe tests for bradykinesia.
- Assessment and management of parkinsonism.
- Parkinsonism gait.
- Functional Rating Scale in Parkinsonism.

6

Peripheral Nerve Injuries

A single peripheral nerve is composed of many nerve fibers or axons which are arranged in groups called as fascicle. The majority of nerve volume is composed of connective tissue and not axons although the amount of connective tissue differs from nerve to nerve and at different distance. These connective tissue consists of the endoneurium which covers a single axon. The perineurium which covers the entire fascicle. The interfascicular epineurium that separates the fascicle from each other and then the outer most covering of the peripheral nerve called as the epineurium (Fig. 6.1).

The connective tissue layer helps in protecting and providing nutrition to the enclosed nerve fibers. External to the epineurium is a transparent thin layer of mesoneurium which serves to secure nerve to adjacent structures such as tendons, vessels, muscles and fascial planes.

The neural structure is comprised of axons and their accompanying Schwann cells. Even the neural fibers and their Schwann cells are surrounded by collagen fibrils to bring about some degree of condensation. Schwann cells are placed along the longitudinal extent of the axon. In between the Schwann cells there is the node of Ranvier which causes salutatory conduction of impulse. The nerve fibers are of two types, the large fibers and the smaller fibers. The larger fibers are more myelinated and concerned with muscles, touch, pressure and some pain. The smaller diameter fiber concerned with autonomic and most pain.

CLASSIFICATION

There are two classifications of PNI which were put forth by Seddom and Sutherland. The *Seddom* classification of PNI is neurapraxia, axonotmesis and neurotmesis.

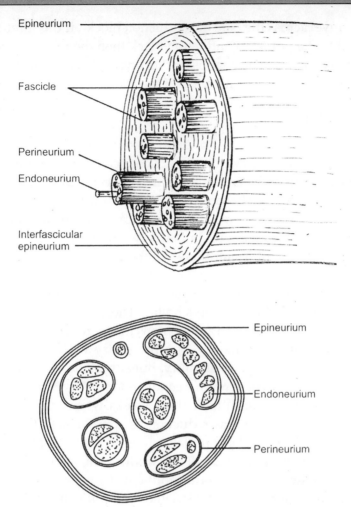

Fig. 6.1: Transverse section of a peripheral nerve

Neurapraxia

In this there is a block in the conduction of impulse down the nerve fiber and recovery takes place without wallerian degeneration. This is probably a biochemical lesion caused by a concussion or shock like injury to the nerve fiber. In case of nerve trunk, neurapraxia is usually brought by compression or stretch, relatively mild blunt blow and low velocity missile injuries close to the nerve, e.g. Saturday night palsy, peroneal palsy due to prolonged cross legged sitting.

Stimulation of the nerve proximal to the site of block will not be able to produce a response distal to the site of lesion as the impulse fail to travel across the "site of conduction block". If the stimulation is distal to the point of conduction block then the response will be obtained distally. The prognosis of this type of nerve injury is very good as there is no degeneration of the axon.

Axonotmesis

In axonetmesis there is loss of relative continuity of the axon with its myelin sheath but with an intact connective tissue framework hence wallerian degeneration is a must to occur. During the initial stage of axonotmesis it become very difficult to differentiate between neurapraxia and axonotmesis both clinically and through electro-physiological investigations. But after two weeks of nerve injury in axonotmesis type of lesion there will be presence of spontaneous activity like either fibrillation potential or denervation potential. These spontaneous activity are due to an increased hypersensitivity of the motor end plate to acetylcholine. There is loss of motor, sen-sory and in some cases even autonomous function. Nerve conduction velocity testing immediately after the injury will show reduced conduction across the site of injury. But stimulation below the site of injury will show a near normal conduction velocity but these keeps reducing gradually until after three weeks when the conduction velocity will show a gross reduction as compared to the normal value. After three weeks stimulation on the nerve trunk proximal or distal to the site of lesion will not produce any response. There is also retrograde degeneration up to the proximal node of Ranvier which further delays the recovery. Recovery following axonotmesis strictly depends upon the rate and extent of regeneration. Proximal lesion grow little faster than distal lesion. If the lesion is proximal then the regeneration may be at a rate of 2 to 3 mm per day but if the lesion is distal then it takes place at a rate of 1 to 1.5 mm per day. As more and more regenerating fibres cross the point of lesion recording of nerve action potential across the site of lesion becomes possible but the amplitude of the potential will be small initially but progressively comes towards normal value as the proportion of regenerating fibers in the nerve trunk increases. Recovery following a axonotmesis becomes evident through electrophysiological testing much before clinical examination. Potential of recovery is always better in axonotmesis as compared to neurotmesis mainly due to the intact connective tissue framework in the former.

Neurotmesis

Injuries which cause nerve contusion, severe stretch or laceration produce neurotmesis in which not only the axon but even the investing connective tissue framework gets disrupted and lose their continuity. Example of a neurotmesis is nerve transection because in this both the axon and the connective tissue loose its continuity. However, not all type of neurotmesis involve complete transection of the nerve trunk but rather internal disruption of the architecture of the nerve sufficient to involve perineurium and endoneurium as well as axons and their coverings. EMG findings are same as that of axonotmesis. In the initial stage of injury, nerve conduction velocity testing in complete neurapraxia and neurotmesis gives a relative similar picture causing confusion in the diagnosis. However if the NCV study is repeated after 2 to 3 weeks of injury, stimulation proximal to the site of lesion and recording distally will not produce any response but on stimulating distally nerve with complete neurapraxia will show a near normal response whereas in complete neurotmesis there will be gross decrease in the conduction velocity. Spontaneous reversal of these changes and recovery are unlikely to occur because regenerating axons become mixed in a swirl of regenerating fibroblasts and collagen producing a disorganized repair site or neuroma. Although the axons may reach the distal stump in great number in neurotmesis but they often fail to find their earlier pathways and may even behave as free nerve ending causing abnormal sensory manifestation in the patient. Most importantly because of endoneurial proliferation and contraction of the distal nerve sheath they may fail to regain sufficient axonal diameter and myelination to produce functional regeneration even if they do reach proper destinations.

Sutherlands on the other hand classified nerve injury into five grades which are as follows (Fig. 6.2):

Grade I or first degree nerve injury which corresponds to a neurapraxia.

Grade II or second degree injury involves loss of axon continuity with preservation of endoneurium and fascicular structure.

Grade III or third degree injury is a mixed axonotmetic– neurotmetic type of injury wherein both axons and endoneurium are damaged but most of the perineurium and therefore the fascicular structures is maintained.

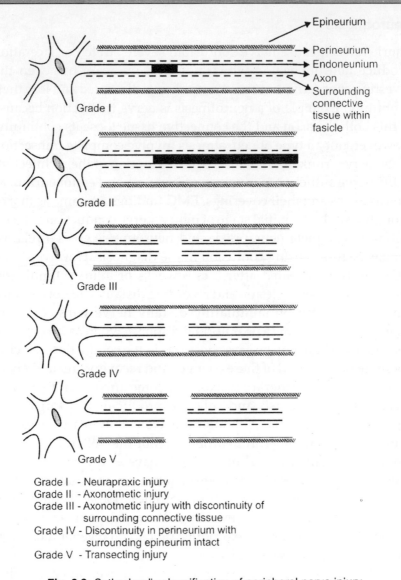

Grade I   - Neurapraxic injury
Grade II   - Axonotmetic injury
Grade III - Axonotmetic injury with discontinuity of
             surrounding connective tissue
Grade IV   - Discontinuity in perineurium with
             surrounding epineurim intact
Grade V   - Transecting injury

Fig. 6.2: Sutherland's classification of peripheral nerve injury

Grade IV or fourth degree injury involves loss of axons, endo-neurium, perineurium with absence of fascicular structure. The continuity of the nerve trunk is maintained only by the intact epineurium.

Grade V or fifth degree nerve injury which involves a complete transection of the nerve trunk and so a complete neurotmesis by definition.

ASSESSMENT OF PHERIPHERAL NERVE INJURY

After collecting the demographic information, chief complain, history from the patient, one should proceed with the evaluation in the following manner:

Observation

Attitude of the part (presence of wrist drop, claw hand etc) wasting, trophic changes in the skin (indicates either prolonged inactivity or involvement of fiber in the peripheral nerve regulating autonomic function.), pilomotor response and edema.

Examination

Sensory

The therapist may evaluate the sensory function along the cutaneous distribution of that peripheral nerve. Thus, interpretation of the sensory dysfunctions is also with respect to the distribution of the peripheral nerve and not dermatomically.

Reflexes

The deep and superficial reflexes should be checked only if the particular nerve or its muscular supply are involved in the reflex arc for any specific reflex. Thus deep tendon jerk should be tested for musculocutaneous nerve involvement (biceps is supplied by musculocutaneous nerve) but can be avoided for ulnar nerve injury.

Tone

Quick passive movement is done to examine tone. In PNI the patient has hypotonicity or atonicity.

MMT

Individual MMT is to be done; the therapist should also have adequate knowledge about the types of trick movements to be noticed in patient with weakness or paralysis because otherwise the grading may be completely wrong.

Sweat Function Test

This is one of the ways to check out for involvement of autonomous function in peripheral nerve injury. There are four types of sweat function test that may be used commonly.

The Q-Sweat (Quantitative Sweat Measurement System) quantifies human skin sweat output. This patented device precisely measures sweat rate and volume via a closed chamber that is affixed to the skin and displays the data in real time in an easy-to-read, Windows-based graphical user interface.

Ninhydrin Test

Ninhydrin powder is sprayed over the skin. When this powder comes in contact with the skin it changes it's color. If the color does not change then it means the area does not have sweat function. (To stimulate sweating the patient may be given an atmosphere that will stimulate sweat reaction).

Chinizarin Start Test

Prepare dry powder mixture of quinizarin (Chinizarin) sodium 35 g, sodium carbonate 30 g, and rice starch 30 g. Dust the reddish-grey powder over skin to be tested and place under heat cradle for 15 to 45 minutes. The powder will change its color when comes in contact with sweat.

Galvanic Skin Resistance Test

Sweating will decrease the skin resistance and will facilitate flow of current through skin, thus if the resistance offered by skin surface is more than the other areas in the body then it can be interpreted that there is sweat dysfunction which is contributing towards the increased skin resistance.

Investigations

SDC should be done periodically. It may show a normal response till wallerian degeneration is complete but later will show signs of denervation. EMG should be done and will show a typical neurogenic presentation. NCV will show decrease conduction velocity across the lesion but proper interpretation is necessary to differentiate between neurapraxia, axonotemeis and neurotemesis. F latency can be done to confirm proximal lesion to the motor axon.

MANAGEMENT FOR PHERIPHERAL NERVE INJURY

Acute Stage

This is a stage of total paralysis. Hence, the main aim of the management will be as under:

To Maintain the Properties of the Muscle

This can be achieved by stimulating paralyzed muscles using interrupted galvanic current. Galvanic current can stimulate denervated muscle as they are of longer pulse duration. Artificially contracting muscles will ensure a proper blood supply as well as help in maintenance of excitation, contraction and coupling. Faradic current cannot be used for these purposes as it is of shorter pulse duration and hence does not stimulate denervated muscles.

To Maintain Joint Range of Motion

Passive range of motion is giving to the paralyzed area so that the joint range of motion can be maintained. The flexibility of the muscles can also be maintained by gentle sustained stretch.

To Prevent any Abnormal Attitude of the Affected Part

Splinting is necessary for the purpose of giving a functional position and also to prevent overstretching of the affected muscles.

To Maintain the Skin Texture

This management is very essential while treating patients with trophic skin changes. The affected area should be kept supple by applying some moisturizer or oil so that skin breakdown can be prevented.

Care of Anesthetic Hand or Foot

The involved part should be inspected regularly for some wounds, or skin color changes. In case of any wound immediate antiseptic precaution should be taken. The patient should be asked to avoid extreme temperatures. Protective gloves may be used for hand to prevent injury by sharp objects. Soft shoes, preferably with toe windows may be worn to protect the foot. The skin should be kept moist but not wet. Proper hygienic measures should be taken to prevent any infection to the affected area.

Prevention of Edema

This is possible in cases of gross paralysis of the upper or lower limb like a brachial plexus or sciatic nerve injury respectively. Odema occurs due to gravity dependent position of limb coupled with lack of muscular tone hence elastocrepe bandage and elevation is given to prevent edema

Consistent Monitoring

The patient should be monitored by the therapist quite regularly for checking any deterioration or improvement in the condition. SDC is done every week to note the signs of innervations.

Recovery Stage

In this stage innervation has started and the muscle begins to show active contraction. Thus the aim of treatment will be as under:

Muscle Reeducation

Once the MMT grade is I or if the SDC is showing signs of innervations then faradic reeducation should be given to the muscle. In this treatment Faradic current is used to produce the action of a muscle and the patient is asked to put in voluntary effort along with the current. The intensity of the current is slowly decreased during the subsequent session so that the patient will be able to perform the action without any assistance.

Combination of Faradic Re-education and Biofeedback

This method is very effective to bring about muscle reeducation as the biofeedback helps the patient to understand the outcome of his effort and thus can motivate the patient to contribute more

Strengthening

Once the muscle power has reached MMT grade 2 then strengthening exercises can be started in gravity eliminated plane or inclined plane till the power reaches 3. Reeducation board or table is helpful in gradually changing the muscle work from a gravity eliminated plane to against gravity. Once the muscle power reaches grade 3 then resisted exercises can be given manually or with springs, pulleys, hydrotherapy etc.

Functional Retraining

Although the muscle may appears to be strengthened to the maximum grade, but it is essential to incorporate functional activity into the rehabilitation program. This is necessary because an increase in strength of a muscle for one activity does not necessarily guarantee efficient performance for other activity. Thus for hand various gripping activities and for lower limbs activities like level walking, staircase climbing etc needs to be given. *It should be noted that the therapist should wait for adequate time for recovery to take place that can be calculated considering the rate of regeneration (1mm per day on an average) and the site of lesion. However once the patient does not recover in the predicted time then based on various investigation and evaluation he may be sent for plastic surgery intervention. This is essential to give some functional independence to the patient. These treatment principles can be applied for all the nerves.*

Brachial Plexus Injury (Fig. 6.3)

- Traction injury
- Penetrating wounds
- Stab wounds or gun shot wounds
- Vehicular accidents
- Birth injuries
- Fracture dislocation of the scapula, clavicle or upper part of the humerus
- Shoulder girdle neuritis
- An unusually large cervical rib
- Malignancy of the cervical lymph nodes
- Congenital abnormality of the cervical spine like the Klippel Fail syndrome
- Apical lung tumors.

Types

Brachial plexus injury is classified mainly base upon the site of injury as preganglionic, postganglionic and total plexus injury.

Preganglionic injury is caused due to avulsion of the roots from the spinal cord. This type of lesion produces both sensory and motor loss. As in preganglionic lesion the dorsal root ganglion is separated from the spinal cord wallerian degeneration doesn't take place in the sensory axon even though the patient has peripheral anesthesia. Axon reflex remains intact in the initial stage of the injury. Conduction velocity of the sensory axon remains intact but that of the motor axon remains lost. The prognosis of this type of injury is very poor.

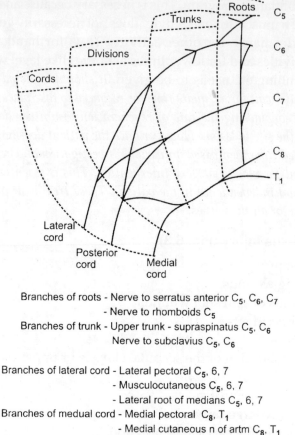

Branches of roots - Nerve to serratus anterior C_5, C_6, C_7
- Nerve to rhomboids C_5
Branches of trunk - Upper trunk - supraspinatus C_5, C_6
Nerve to subclavius C_5, C_6

Branches of lateral cord - Lateral pectoral C_5, 6, 7
- Musculocutaneous C_5, 6, 7
- Lateral root of medians C_5, 6, 7
Branches of medual cord - Medial pectoral C_8, T_1
- Medial cutaneous n of artm C_8, T_1
- Medial cutaneous N of forearm C_8, T_1
- Ulnar C_8 and T_1
- Medial root of median C_8, T_1
Branches of posterior cord - Upper subscapular C_5, 6
- Nerve to latissimus dorsi C_6, C_7, C_8
- Lower subscapular C_5, C_6
- Axillary C_5, C_6
- Radial nerve C_5, C_6, C_7, C_8, T_1

Fig. 6.3: Brachial plexus injury

Postganglionic lesions are the one in which the lesion is distal to the dorsal root ganglion. There is sensory and motor loss. The axon reflex is also lost. Conduction velocity of both the sensory axon and motor axon is affected. As the dorsal root ganglion is not in contact with the remaining portion of the axon, wallerian degeneration is a must and hence such type of injury has a good prognosis.

Total plexus injury is the one in which the lesion is very close to the vertebral column. This type of brachial plexus injury is very rare. All the muscles supplied by the brachial plexus are paralyzed and even the cervical sympathetic is involved. However if the plexus is involved at the level of the trunk then certain muscles like the rhomboids, serratus anterior, spinalis and pectorals may be spared. Appreciation of touch, pain, thermal sensation is lost over the hand, forearm and the lower third of the upper arm. Joint position sensitivity is lost in the fingers. Tendon reflexes in the upper limb is lost.

ERB'S PALSY

Injury to the upper trunk originating from C5 and C6 nerve roots or injury to the C5 and C6 nerve root causes Erb- Duchenne palsy.

Causes

- Indirect injury
- Vacuum delivery
- Pressure on the supraclavicular area
- During anesthesia
- Injection of foreign vaccines and serum.

Signs and Symptoms

Sensory

There is loss of sensation in the area of deltoid insertion and lateral aspect of the forearm and hand.

Motor

The muscle that will be totally paralyzed are the deltoid, biceps, brachia, brachialis, brachioradialis, supraspinatus, infraspinatus, teres minor, rhomboids and supinator. The muscles that will not be totally paralyzed but will be just weak are triceps, latissimus dorsi, serratus anterior, pectoralis major and extensor carpi radialis.

Reflexes

Biceps and brachioradialis jerks are affected.

Deformity

The patient will exhibit a deformity which is usually called as policeman's tip or waiter's tip. This deformity consists of extension, adduction, internal rotation at the shoulder, extension at the elbow, pronation and flexion at the wrist and fingers.

Functional Disability

All the activities of daily living which involves flexion movement at the shoulder and the elbow will be lost. Thus the patient will have difficulty in eating, combing, washing, dressing, reaching out and other similar activities.

Treatment

The treatment comprises of:
- IG stimulation to maintain the muscles property.
- Passive movement and stretching to prevent any joint contracture or deformity.
- Care of edema is very necessary as the hand is always in dependent position with respect to the gravity hence more chances of developing edema.
- Massage may be given to maintain the circulation and prevent any trophic changes.
- Splint that is given is aimed at maintaining the shoulder in the functional position. Two splints commonly used are aeroplane splint and cheese splint. Both the splints prevents contracture of adductors and internal rotators. These splints also prevents any chances of shoulder dislocation.

It should be noted that the prognosis of Erb's palsy is much better than the Klumpke's palsy as the distal that need to be covered by the axon to reach the end organ is very short.
- Strengtheing exercises once recovery starts.

KLUMPKE'S PALSY

Any lesion to the lower trunk of brachial plexus or to C8, T1 roots of the spinal cord.

Causes

- Breech delivery
- Traction and fall in the abducted arm
- Operation in the axilla
- Tumor in the apical lobe of the lung
- Enlarged cervical rib.

Signs and Symptoms

Sensory

There will be loss of sensation over the medial aspect of the arm, forearm, hand and hypothenar eminence.

Motor

There will be paralysis of all the intrinsics of the hand along with wrist and finger flexors.

Deformity

The patient will have claw hand deformity.

Functional Disability

As the patient will lack intrinsic plus grip or lubrical grip, the patient's power grip is very inefficient. The skin will become very dry, scaly and the nails will become brittle.

Treatment

- Stimulation
- Passive movements
- Massage
- Splintage: Knuckle bender splint is given for the hand.
- Strengthening exercises once the nerve gets innervated.

RADIAL NERVE INJURY (Fig. 6.4)

Causes

Axilla

- Crutch palsy
- Deep penetrating injury in the axilla
- Diphtheria involving the radial nerve in the axilla
- Lead poisoning which generally causes bilateral involvement of the radial nerve
- Saturday night palsy.

Upper Arm

- Tourniquet's palsy involving all three nerves
- Fracture shaft humerus

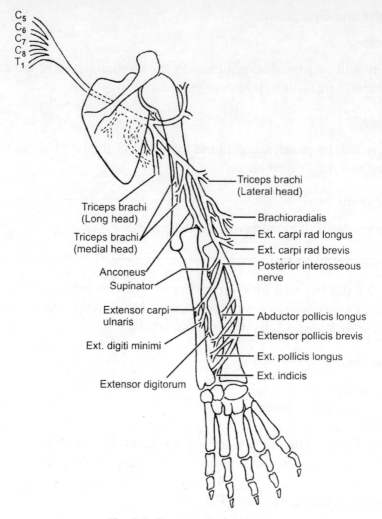

Fig. 6.4: Course of radial nerve

- Injection palsy
- Gun shot or glass cut injury
- Supracondylar palsy
- Radial nerve can be compressed under the fibrous arch formed by the triceps muscle just 2 cm below the deltoid insertion. The nerve gets compressed due to vigorous contraction of the triceps muscles.

At the Elbow

- Tennis elbow
- Inflammation of the common extensor tendon may heal by fibrosis and compress the radial nerve
- Fracture of the upper end of radius and ulna
- Direct blow to the posterior interosseous nerve
- A fibrous arch covers the posterior interosseous nerve as its passes through the supinator muscles and can gets compressed during forceful contraction of the muscles.
- Two layers of supinator can also compress the nerve against the aponeurosis of extensor carpi radialis brevis.
- Compression of the posterior interosseus nerve due to ganglia, neoplasm, bursae, VIC and fibrosis after trauma.

Signs and Symptoms

Sensory

There will be loss of sensation over the following areas depending upon the level of lesion.
- Posterior part of the upper arm
- Lower lateral part of the arm
- Posterior part of the forearm
- Posterior part of the hand and the fingers up to the nail beds.

The autonomous zone for the radial nerve is the first web space. When the posterior interosseous nerve only is involved then the patient will not have anesthesia of the autonomous zone as the posterior interosseous nerve is a purely motor nerve.

Motor Loss

The following muscles will be involved depending upon the level of lesion:
- Triceps, brachioradialis, extensor carpi radialis longus and brevis, extensor carpi ulnaris, extensor digitorum, extensor digiti minimi, supinator, anconeus, abductor pollicies longus, extensor pollicies longus and brevis, extensor indicis.
- Not all the muscles will be involved in all the cases of radial nerve palsy. It all depends upon the site of radial nerve injury. Careful examination of muscle power hence becomes an important tool to detect the level of the nerve injury.

Reflexes

The triceps and brachioradialis jerk will be depressed or absent depending upon the level of lesion.

Deformity

Wrist drop in which the wrist is held in some 45 degree of palmar flexion due to the overaction of the wrist flexors unopposed by their antagonist which is the paralyzed wrist extensors. The thumb is held in palmar abduction and slight flexion due to the unopposed action of the short flexor and short abductor. The metacarpophalangeal joints are held in about 30 degree of flexion due to the unopposed action of the lumbricals, as the extensor digitorum is paralyzed. There is only slight flexion at the interphalangeal joints as the interossei extend these joints and are unaffected, the slight flexion in that due to the wrist and metacarpophalangeal joints taking up a position of flexion which automatically results in slight flexion at the proximal and distal interphalangeal joints.

Attempts to perform pure ulnar deviation results in vigorous flexion along with ulnar deviation as there is unopposed action of the flexor carpi ulnaris which is not balanced by the paralyzed extensor carpi ulnaris.

Functional disability: The patient generally will have a poor grip due to lack of wrist extensor as fixator and cannot put objects like glasses or cups flat on the table.

Common Trick Movements

- As the wrist extensors are paralyzed the patient may attempts to perform wrist extension by forcefully contraction and then relaxation giving an impression of wrist extension. This type of trick movement is *Rebound phenomena.*
- To bring about extension of the MCP joint, in absence of paralyzed extensor digitorum, the dorsal interossei may bring about finger extension but the fingers will have the tendency to go into abduction as well.
- Extension of DIP of the thumb is done by rebound phenomena where the flexor pollicies longus forcefully contract and relax giving rise to false impression of extensor pollicies longus action.
- Extensor carpi radialis is the first muscles to recover in radial nerve palsy so attempted dorsiflexion results in a radial deviation

because the extensor carpi ulnaris is still paralyzed and hence cannot balance. The early sign of recovery of the extensor carpi ulnaris is reduced tendency of the wrist to go into radial deviation.

- Extension of the DIP of the thumb is also possible due to accessory insertion of abductor pollicies brevis hence every time the patient does abduction which is perpendicular to the palm. There will be extension of the DIP of the thumb.
- Due to paralysis of triceps the patient may use gravitational force to bring about elbow extension.

Treatment

Conservative management(Figs 6.5 and 6.6, Plate 4)

Homeostasis of the involved extremity must be established before reconstruction. The patient must maintain a full range of passive motion in all the joints of the hand and wrist. The therapist must prevent any contracture giving particular attention to the thumb—index web. Individualized treatment may include a dynamic splint. The main aim behind giving splintage is to prevent wrist flexion as well to give functional position of wrist extension so that the patient can use his long flexors and intrinsic effectively to perform various activities of daily living. Also the splint should be able to prevent adductor pollicies and pronator contracture.

The splints usually given is either static or dynamic splints. The static splints used are either cock up splint with a ventral or dorsal support or a Robert Jones splints which keeps the wrist and finger in extension.

The dynamic splints used are either cockup splints with extensor out triggers or cockup splint with reverse knuckle bender.

The other conservative physiotherapy managements and its aim remains same as described in the initial part of this chapter.

Surgical treatment

The requirement for restoration of wrist and hand function are:
- Wrist extension
- Finger metacarpophalangeal extension
- Thumb extension
- Stability of the carpometacarpal joints of the thumb.

Loss of forearm supination secondary to loss of supinator muscle is inconsequential in the presence of a normal biceps brachii. There is loss of gross grip strength related to radial palsy because wrist extension is necessary to provide stability and to allow full excursion of the digital flexors. Precision pinch is weak when the base of the thumb is unstable due to paralyzed of the abductor pollicies longus.

Tendon transfer done is as follows

- Pronator Teres is transferred for restoration of extension of the wrist thereby substituting for the loss of ECRL and ECRB. Thus after transfer the pronator teres will act as a wrist extensor but will still perform pronator action. After the anastomosis the wrist should rest in 30 degree of extension against gravity. If the tension becomes too much the functional wrist flexion will become impossible.

- For gaining thumb stability it is desirable to repower the abductor pollicies longus. Without this stability, strong pinch is impaired and incomplete abduction of the first metacarpophalangeal joint will cause some awkwardness during fine precision activity. The flexor carpi radialis tendon can be split and the radial half of the tendon transferred to the abductor pollicies longus tendon or the Palmaris longus tendon is transferred to the extensor pollicies brevis tendon.

- Elbow extension: Trauma to the upper extremity in isolated radial palsy usually is distal to the branches to the triceps muscle in the upper arm. Posterior deltoid to triceps transfer is most preferable for elbow extension activity which is such an important action for weight bearing function of the upper limb.

- Finger extension: Flexor carpi ulnaris to long finger extensor transfer is the most preferable for restoring finger extension.

Robert Jones transfer is as under:

- Pronator Teres for ECRL and ECRB
- FCU for ED
- FCR for EPL/EPB/APL

As following the transfer the wrist was rendered unstable as no flexors were left on the flexors aspect. Therefore there was a modification known as Zachary's modification where FDS of the ring finger or Palmaris longus was used for EPL/EPB/APL.

Preoperatively the strength of the donor muscles should always be strengthened to the maximum.

Postoperative physiotherapy management: In operating room, a double sugar tong splint is applied which immobilizes the forearm in 30 degree of pronation, the wrist in 40-45 degree of extension, the metacarpophalangeal joint in 0 degree of extension and the thumb in maximum extension and abduction. The first splint extends beyond the proximal interphalangeal joints, which are volarly supported in 45 degree of flexion. This splint is removed in 48 hours and a long arm cast is applied. The proximal interphalangeal joints are free but all other joints are immobilized as noted above.

After 5 weeks of surgery the patient is removed from rigid immobilization and placed in a spring action cockup splint to obtain independent action for wrist and finger extension. A planned exercise program will use synergistic movements.

Following tendon transfer, after 3 weeks faradic reeducation is started. In order to train the muscle for its new action one must resist the original action of the muscle because in the initial stages the transferred muscle will have the tendency to perform the original action. In case of the transferred pronator teres, during the initial stages of faradic reeducation, the forearm tends to go into pronation which needs to inhibited. On inhibition the wrist will go into extension that has to be encouraged. Once the muscle learn the new action it has to be strengthened by various strengthening techniques and thereby it should be used for various functions.

MEDIAN NERVE INJURY (Fig. 6.7)

Median nerve can be involved anywhere along the course:

Axilla

- Axillary aneurysm
- Traction injury

Arm

Penetrating injury

Elbow

- Penetrating injury
- Hansen's disease
- Tourniquet's palsy
- Golfer's elbow
- Supracondylar fracture

Forearm

- Pronator teres syndrome; A fibrous band that travels between the deep and superficial head of the pronator teres can compress

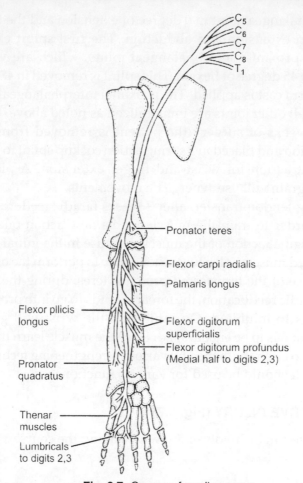

C_5
C_6
C_7
C_8
T_1

Pronator teres

Flexor carpi radialis

Palmaris longus

Flexor pllicis longus

Flexor digitorum superficialis

Flexor digitorum profundus (Medial half to digits 2,3)

Pronator quadratus

Thenar muscles

Lumbricals to digits 2,3

Fig. 6.7: Course of median nerve

the median nerve due to over use or violent contraction of the muscle.

- A fibrous arch which originates just proximal to the origin of the flexor digitorum superficialis can compress the median nerve causing selected paralysis of FDS and FDP.
- Volkmann's ischemic contracture.

Wrist

- Glass cut injury can cause isolated involvement of the median nerve or alongwith the ulnar nerve.
- Carpal tunnel syndrome.

Anterior interosseous nerve can get involved due to fracture or laceration of the forearm. It can be compressed by the flexor digitorum superficialis or pronator teres. It can also be involved due to VIC or thrombosis of the ulnar collateral vessels.

Signs and Symptoms

Sensory

There will be loss of sensation over the volar aspect of lateral 3½ fingers up to the distal phalanx on the dorsal side, skin overlying the thenar eminence. The autonomous zone for the median nerve is the pulp of the thumb.

Motor

The muscles supplied by the median nerve namely the pronator teres, flexor carpi radialis, flexor digitorum superficialis, palmaris longus, flexor digitorum profundus(the lateral half), pronatus quadratus, flexor pollicis longus, thenar muscles, the first and second lumbricals.

Deformity

The deformity seen in median nerve palsy are as follows depending upon the site and extent of lesion.
- The commonest deformity seen is ape hand or monkey hand which occurs due to flattening of the thenar eminence, lack of opposition of the thumb because of which the thumb is held beside the index finger due to over action of the adductor pollicis and extensor pollicis longus.
- Partial claw hand occurs due to paralysis of the first and second lumbricals due to which there is unopposed action of the extensor digitorum giving rise to hyperextension of the metacarpophalangeal joint of the index and middle finger alongwith flexion of the interphalangeal joint of these fingers. With lesion at the wrist the interphalangeal flexion will increase due to increased activity of flexor digitorum superficialis and profundus as they will be spared.
- Pointing index finger: When there is a higher lesion involving even the long flexors of the hand, on asking to make a fist the index finger will point forward. This happens because when the patient attempts to make a fist, the profundus tendon of the ring finger will pull the middle finger into partial flexion leaving the index finger in extension and pointing forward.
- When patient with anterior interosseous nerve palsy is asked to make a tip to tip pinch using the index and the thumb then due

to paralysis of the flexor digitorum profundus and flexor pollicis longus the tip to tip pinch will show a tear drop appearance instead of 'O'.

Functional disability: Most of the patient with median nerve palsy will be having difficulty in holding both big and small object. Their activity with the involved hand is generally clumpsy because they cannot hold object confidentially in their hand nor they can appreciate the sensation of the object unless and until they see the object.

Trick movements: Common trick movement which can be expected in patient's with median nerve injury are as follows:
- Due to paralysis of pronator teres the patient will try to pronate with the help of brachioradialis along with internal rotation of the arm.
- To perform radial deviation the patient substitutes with the help of extensor carpi radialis and to perform wrist flexion, he will use the flexor carpi ulnaris.
- In the absence of FPL, the patient may perform flexion of the distal interphalangeal joint by rebound phenomena using a strong contraction of the extensor pollicis longus and suddenly relaxing.
- To perform opposition action the patient uses abductor pollicis longus and then let the thumb fall toward the palm due to the force of gravity.
  The first sign of recovery of median nerve following its lesion in the wrist will be the ability of the thumb to rotate when the thumb is supported in slight amount of palmar abduction and flexion.

Treatment

Conservative physiotherapy management:
- Passive movement to the wrist and fingers to keep the parts mobile
- Gentle stretching of the long flexors to prevent any form of tightness
- IG stimulation to all the muscles supplied by the median nerve
- Care of the anaesthetic hand
- Splints: Opposition splints are given to maintain the thumb in opposition and also to prevent contracture of the first web space.

The two types of splints which are commonly given are C- bar and cockup splints. The C- bar can be made up of aluminium, orthoplast and plaster of Paris. This is used to maintain the first web space and is held in place with the help of 3 velcro straps one over the index finger, one over the thumb and one at the deepest part of the first web space (Fig 6.9 B and 6.9C).

Cock up splint with an opposition out trigger is also used to maintain the thumb in opposition.

Surgical management: The basic requirement for hand function in median nerve injury consist of the following component.

- Thumb abduction to perform opposition
- Flexion across the metacarpophalangeal joint of the thumb
- Flexion of the index and middle finger
- Sensation over the thenar eminence and pulp of the thumb.

In addition to the above even pronation of the forearm becomes quite essential when there is a lesion higher up.

The preferable surgical procedure is a tendon transfer and the commonest types of tendon transfer for median nerve injury is as follows:

- Restoration of thumb opposition is done by transferring the flexor digitorum superficialis of the ring finger which is detached from its insertion wound around the flexor carpi ulnaris tendon and inserted to the insertion of abductor pollicis brevis. Following surgery, the thumb is immobilized in opposition position for three weeks in POP after this an opposition splint can be given for another 6 weeks during which physiotherapy treatment involving reeducation of the transferred tendon is done along the same line.
- Flexion of DIP of the thumb can be achieved by detaching brachioradialis from its insertion and attaching it along with the flexor pollicis longus. Extensor digiti minimi can also be used.
- Flexion of the index and middle finger can be achieved by slitting the tendon of flexor digitorum profundus of the ring and little finger and attaching them to the middle and index finger so that the ulnar portion of the nerve can pull the fingers into flexion.
- In very rare cases biceps tendon may be transferred to perform pronation.

In all the above cases faradic reeducation may be started after 3 weeks.

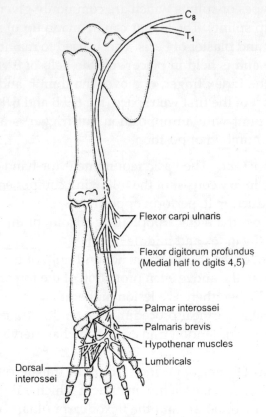

Fig. 6.8: Course of ulnar nerve

Intermetacarpal blocks may also be given between the first and second metacarpal to maintain the first web space permanently.

ULNAR NERVE INJURY (Fig. 6.8)

Causes

At the Cervical Spine

- Prolapse intervertebral disc
- Osteophyte due to cervical spondylosis
- Rheumatoid diseases of the cervical spine

At the Base of the Neck

- Cervical rib
- Thoracic outlet syndrome
- Scalenus anticus syndrome

At the Axilla

Crutch palsy.

Arm

- Tourniquet palsy
- Fracture of the supracondylar region of humerus
- Hansen's disease.

Elbow

- Cubitus valgus causing Tardy ulnar nerve palsy: At the elbow the ulnar nerve passes through a tunnel the roof of which is formed by a fibrous arch. This arch becomes tight during elbow flexion as the floor of the capsule bulges out. In cubitus valgus the floor is already elevated which increases the compression on the ulnar nerve. Initially this leads to only conduction block but later to degeneration.
- Dislocation of the elbow.
- Fracture of the medial epicondyle of the humerus.
- Hansen's disease.

At the Forearm

- Volkmann's ischemic contracture
- Tight plaster

At the Wrist

- Glass cut injury
- Compression of the ulnar nerve as it passes through the canal of Guyon. The medial border of this canal is formed by the tendon of flexor carpi ulnaris and pisiform bone. The floor of the canal is formed by the flexor retinaculum and the roof is formed by the superficial part of the flexor retinaculum.
- Fracture of the carpus bone
- Tumors
- Osteoarthritis.

Signs and Symptoms

Sensory Loss

The patient will have loss of sensation on the skin overlying the hypothenar eminence, the medial 1½ finger up to the nail beds.

Motor Loss

The muscles that will be affected are flexor carpi ulnaris, medial half of the flexor digitorum profundus, the hypothenar muscles, medial two lumbricals, the adductor pollicis, and the interossei.

Deformity

The patient will exhibit classical claw hand deformity where there is hyperextension of the metacarpophalangeal joint of the ring and little finger to about 30 degrees, due to over action of the extensor digitorum and extensor digiti minimi. The interphalangeal joint of these two fingers will be held in flexion, the proximal interphalangeal joint is held at about 25 degrees of flexion. The distal interphalangeal joint may be flexed or extended depending upon the site of injury to the ulnar nerve. If the ulnar nerve is involved at the wrist there will be about 10 to 15 degrees of flexion at the distal interphalangeal joint due to over action of the flexor digitorum profundus but if the lesion is at the elbow then there will be paralysis of even the profundus causing reduced flexion at the distal interphalangeal joint.

Ulnar paradox: With lesion at the elbow there is reduced flexion at the distal interphalangeal joint due to paralysis of flexor digitorum profundus. With reinnervation the flexion at the DIP joint will increase giving an appearance of increase deformity although this is a prognostic sign.

Functional Disability

- The patient will lack intrinsic plus position or lumbrical grip
- Power grip is more affected due to lack of the elevation of the hypothenar eminence, inability of the fingers to wrap around the object and due to the lack of clamping action of the thumb.
- Pinch power reduces
- Spherical grip is lacking due to absence of lateralization of fingers
- Lateral pinch becomes inefficient due to paralyzed adductor pollicis.

Trick Movements

- Due to paralysis of the lumbricals, extension of the interphalangeal joint will be possible only when the metacarpophalangeal joint is supported in flexion.

- Due to paralysis of dorsal interossei, the patient will try to abduct the finger using extensor digitorum which also causes extension of the fingers.
- Adduction of the finger can be brought about by direct substitution using the long flexors of the hand.
- Ulnar deviation can be brought about by extensor carpi ulnaris.
- When the patient is asked to perform wrist flexion, the flexor carpi radialis substitutes pulling the hand into radial deviation. Hence *the first sign of recovery after a ulnar nerve injury at the elbow is reduced tendency to go into radial deviation.*
- In place of adductor pollicis the patient will use flexor pollicis longus this is called as Forment's sign.
- Cocontraction of flexor pollicis longus and extensor pollicis longus nullify their action at the DIP thereby pulling the thumb into adduction.
- **The first sign of recovery following ulnar nerve injury at the wrist is increased abduction attitude of the little finger because the abductor digiti minimi is the first muscle to recover.**

Management

- IG stimulation
- Passive movement and stretching
- Care of anesthetic hand
- *Splintage:* The splint used should be able to keep the metacarpophalangeal joint in flexion and to maintain the interphalangeal joint in extension. Hence a knuckle bender splint is used. This splint consists of a volar support at the metacarpophalangeal joint and two dorsal supports on the proximal phalanx and on the metacarpal bones (Figs 6.9A to C).

Surgical management Tendon transfer surgery are the usual surgical approach practiced in ulnar nerve injury. The commonest tendon transfer done is Paul Brand's transfer where Extensor carpi radialis is detached from its insertion and lengthened by a free tailed graft of plantaris muscle. This is then slit into four, moved through the lumbrical canal and got to the dorsal aspect where it is attached to the extensor aponeurosis.

When there is severe clawing of the hand with wrist flexion, Riordan's technique is used where the flexor carpi radialis is detached from its insertion, lengthened and then inserted in the same way as Brand's surgery.

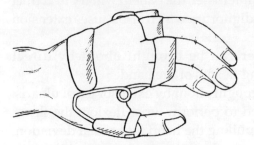

Fig. 6.9A: Splint for combined median and ulnar nerve palsy

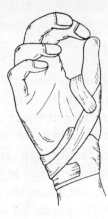

Fig. 6.9B: Dynamic thumb opposition splint for median nerve palsy

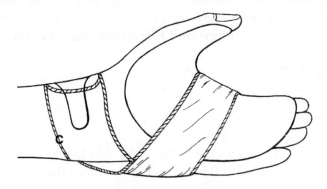

Fig. 6.9C: Bar for median nerve palsy

When there is no habitual flexion of the wrist, Bunnell's surgery may be tried in which case the flexor digitorum of the ring finger is slit into four tendon and then inserted in the same manner as the Brand's surgery.

Postoperative physiotherapy: Following the transfer the fingers are immobilized in lumbrical grip position by POP that is removed after 10 days. After ten days the suture is removed and the plaster is reapplied for 3 more weeks. At the end of 3 weeks the POP is removed and a cylinder POP applied to all the fingers in an attempt to maintain them in extended position. This is kept for another 10 days after which Faradic Re-education may be given to get active lumbrical grip movement. If the patient is not able to achieve it sometimes POP may be reapplied for another 2 to 3 weeks. However, if the clawing is no longer present and if the patient is able to perform the movement actively then strengthening exercises is started. Initially gentle exercises like paper crumpling is given and eventually various power activities can be strengthened. Lastly, dexterity functions can be trained by various pegbo and exercises.

OBTURATOR NERVE INJURY (Fig. 6.10)

Causes

- Dislocation of the hip joint
- Hernia through the obturator foramen
- Prolonged difficult labor
- Compression of the nerve against the wall of the pelvis by any mass such as tumor or foetus
- Pelvic fracture
- Disease or injury to the sacroiliac or hip joints.

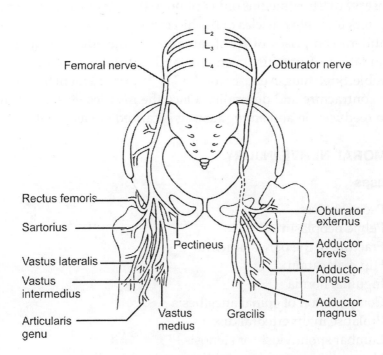

Fig. 6.10: Course of femoral and obturator nerve

Signs and Symptoms

Sensory

There may be loss of sensation over the distal medial aspect of the thigh and medial aspect of the knee.

Motor

The nerve that are paralyzed due to lesion to the anterior division of the obturator nerve are adductor longus, adductor brevis, gracilis and pectineus.

The muscles that are paralyzed due to lesion to the posterior division of the obturator nerve are adductor magnus, obturator externus and occasionally adductor brevis.

Deformity

Due to paralysis of the adductor muscles, the tensor fascia lata overacts hence pulls the hip into flexion, abduction deformity.

Treatment

Conservative treatment is only option in the initial stages as tendon transfers for large muscles of the hip is not possible. Physiotherapy treatment comprises of IG stimulation to the adductor muscles. Stimulation of gracilis, pectineus and obturator externus is not possible. Stretching exercises for the TFL to prevent them from going into contracture and deformity. Once the muscles gets innervated then reeducation and strengthening is carried out as usual.

FEMORAL NERVE INJURY

Causes

- Psoas abscess
- Pelvic neoplasm
- Fracture of the pelvis or femur
- Hip dislocation
- Inguinal hernia
- Complication of spinal anesthesia
- Prolapse intervertebral disc
- Lumbar spondylosis or stenosis
- Neuropathy secondary to diabetes mellitus known as diabetic amyotrophy

- Neurapraxia after hysterectomy or gynecological surgery
- Penetrating wounds of lower abdomen.

Signs and Symptoms

Sensory

There is loss of sensation over the following areas:

a. Anterior division - anterior and medial aspect of the thigh
b. Posterior division – Continuous as the saphenous nerve involving the medial aspect of the leg and foot right up to the ball of the great toe.

The autonomous zone of the femoral nerve is a small area superior and medial to the patella.

Motor

The muscles which are paralyzed due to the lesion of the anterior division are Sartorius and pectineus. The muscles which are paralyzed due to the lesion to the posterior division are rectus femoris, vastus medialis, vastus lateralis and vastus intermedius.

Reflexes

Quadriceps jerk is lost.

Deformity

Genu recurvatum is seen because as the quadriceps is paralyzed the patient will try to lock the knee into hyperextension to get the center of gravity well in front of the knee joint to keep it stable.

Treatment

- Underlying cause must be dealt with
- IG stimulation to the paralyzed muscles
- Passive movements
- Orthosis to correct genu recurvatum. Either anterior knee guard or above knee ankle orthosis.

SCIATIC NERVE INJURY (Fig. 6.11)

Causes

- Penetrating wounds around the pelvis
- Fractures of the pelvis and femur

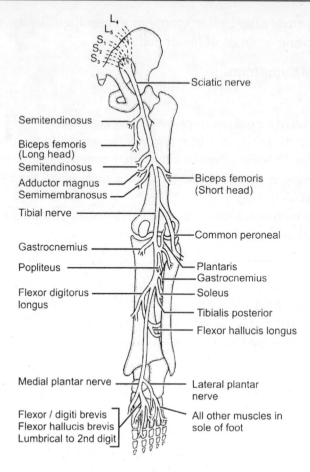

Fig. 6.11: Course of sciatic nerve

- Dislocation of the hip joint
- Badly placed intramuscular injections in the gluteal region
- Compression within the pelvis by a neoplasm or foetal head
- Nerve may undergo entrapment or compression by piriformis muscle as it traverses the sciatic notch.

Signs and Symptoms

Sensory

There will be complete loss of sensation below the knee except for the area that is supplied by the femoral nerve (saphenous nerve).

The autonomous zone for the sciatic nerve is the heel, the skin over the metatarsal head in the sole, the dorsum of the feet as far as medially up to the second metatarsal as well as a small strip of the lateral aspect of the leg.

Motor

The muscles that will be paralyzed are biceps femoris, semi-membranous, semi tendinous, hamstring part of adductor magnus. All the muscles supplied by the tibial and common peroneal which are the branches of the sciatic nerve will also be paralyzed. Thus below the knee all the muscles will be paralyzed.

Deformity

The patient will have flail leg with foot drop. There may be clawing of toes with trophic ulceration. Tropic ulcers develop due to lack of sensation over the foot.

Treatment

- IG stimulation to the paralzsed muscles
- Passive movements
- TA stretching
- Splintage: Night splints such as L splints may be given mainly to prevent foot drop and contractures of the plantar flexors. As the patient has intact quadriceps knee stability is not affected hence below knee caliper such as ankle foot orthosis may be prescribed that will help the patient to be ambulatory in a much comfortable manner
- Padded foot wear or microcellular rubber foot wear
- Metatarsal bar may be given to the foot wear to prevent metatarsal drop
- Care of anaesthetic foot

COMMON PERONEAL NERVE PALSY (Fig. 6.12)

Causes

- Compression of the nerve by tight plaster or a splint
- Fracture of the neck of the fibula
- Fracture dislocation of the head of fibula
- Hansen's disease or leprosy
- Trauma to the knee including rupture of the fibular collateral ligament
- Entrapped, compressed or irritated nerve by fibrous arch as it winds around the neck of fibula

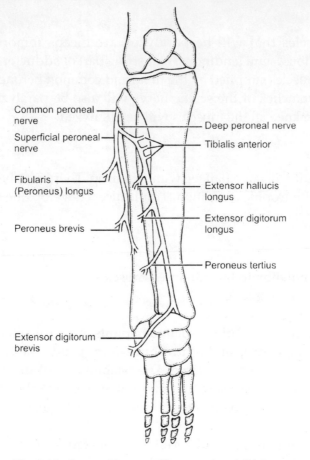

Common peroneal nerve

Superficial peroneal nerve

Fibularis (Peroneus) longus

Peroneus brevis

Extensor digitorum brevis

Deep peroneal nerve

Tibialis anterior

Extensor hallucis longus

Extensor digitorum longus

Peroneus tertius

Fig. 6.12: Course of common peroneal and tibial nerve

- Prolonged immobilization during which the leg lies in external rotation.

Signs and Symptoms

Sensory

Common peroneal nerve by itself is relatively short having only two sensory branches and no motor branches. The loss of sensation is as follows:

a. Skin along the lateral aspect of the knee in the proximal third of the calf (lateral cutaneous sural nerve).

b. Skin over the posterolateral aspect of the calf and over the lateral malleolus, lateral aspect of the foot and fourth and fifth toes (sural nerve).

Common peroneal nerve divides into deep and superficial peroneal nerve.

Deep peroneal nerve palsy leads to loss of sensation over the following areas:

a. Web space between the great and the second toe.
b. Lateral aspect of the dorsum of the great toe.
c. Medial aspect of the dorsum of the second toe.

Superficial peroneal nerve palsy leads to loss of sensation over the following areas:

a. Anterior and lateral aspect of the leg
b. Dorsum of the foot and toes except a small wedge shape area in the web space between the great and the second toe.

Motor

Deep peroneal nerve palsy leads to paralysis of tibialis anterior, extensor hallucis longus, extensor digitorum longus, extensor digitorum brevis and peroneus tertius.

Superficial peroneal palsy leads to paralysis of the peroneus longus and peroneus brevis.

Deformity

Equino varus deformity results due to over action of the posterior compartment muscles and the invertors.

Treatment

Conservative treatment consists of the following:
- IG stimulation of the paralyzed muscles
- Passive movements to maintain the joint range
- Stretching of the Tendoachilles
- Splints or Orthosis: The commonly used orthosis aims to maintain the ankle in neutral position preventing equinous hence either a caliper with dorsiflexion stop or plastic ankle foot orthosis in the form of shoe insert may be prescribed.

Surgical management consists of tendon transfer wherein the tibialis posterior is used to substitute for the lost muscles. The tibialis posterior transfer may be done in two ways:
- Circumtibial route: The tibialis posterior is detached from its insertion circles around tibia and is divided into two clips—one

going to tibialis anterior and extensor hallucies longus whereas the other go to extensor digitorum longus. This procedure is more commonly done but adhesions are likely to occur which are .treated with US, laser and kneading technique.

- Interosseous route: Insertions are the same as above but the transfer is done by piercing the interosseus membrance.

The other surgery which may be carried out involves tendo-Achilles lengthening to get maximum range of dorsiflexion.

Immobilization following tendon transfer can be done in two ways:

- Total period of immobilization is six weeks. For the first three weeks the knee is in flexion and the ankle is in full dorsiflexion. In the next three weeks the knee is kept free but the ankle is still maintained in full dorsiflexion. This method gives a better range of dorsiflexion.
- The ankle is immobilized in full dorsiflexion for a period of six weeks.

Physiotherapy management after surgery: The reeducation of the transferred muscles is classified into two phases:

a. Nonweight-bearing phase: The patient must be shown the method of correct reeducation before surgery the transferred muscle is strengthened by placing the foot on the other thigh and asking the patient to perform inversion. Manual resistance, weight and pulleys can also be used for strengthening. Post-transfer patient may be asked to do the same exercises as above. Faradic reeducation may be given in the initial stages to train the transferred muscle for its new action. Once the new action is learnt biofeedback technique have been very beneficial in faster reeducation.

b. Weight-bearing phase: Take a weighing scale and the patient is asked to bear weight on the affected limb and at the same time carry out dorsiflexion. Initially the patient should take only 10 kg of weight which is indicated by the pointer. This goes on till patient can take more and more weight on the affected limb till he eventually starts taking almost 2/3rd of his body weight (the weight progression is by 10 kg). Then blind fold the patient to see whether the patient knows how much weight is to be taken by the affected limb. This can be checked by the weighing scale.

Then progress to walking on the parallel bars, then even ground, uneven ground and eventually on stairs. The therapist should all the time take care that the patient does not slap the foot on the ground and places it gently. Exercises on the tilt board or vestibular ball has been found to be quite affective in proprioceptive training of the affected foot.

MEDIAL POPLITEAL NERVE (TIBIAL NERVE) INJURY

Causes

- Injection palsy
- Deep penetrating injury to the knee and upper half of the leg
- Dislocation of the knee
- Tarsal tunnel syndrome in which the nerve is entrapped in between the laciniate ligament and the medial surface of the talus, distal to the medial malleolus.

Signs and Symptoms

Sensory

Tibial nerve palsy leads to loss of sensation over the following areas:
- Sole of the foot
- Skin over the medial aspect of the heel

Autonomous zone of the tibial nerve is sole of the foot except the medial border of the foot, lateral surface of the heel and plantar surface of the toes.

Motor

The muscles that are paralyzed are gastrocnemius, plantaris, soleus, flexor hallucis longus, flexor digitorum longus, tibialis posterior and popliteus.

Deformity

The patient will develop talipes calcaneovalgus deformity or dorsiflexion deformity.

Reflexes

The ankle jerk is lost and the plantar reflex may also be inellicitable.

Treatment

Conservative treatment consists of:
• IG stimulation
• Passive movement
• Stretching
• Care of anesthetic foot
• Orthosis: The patient may be prescribed below knee caliper with dorsiflexion stop.

Note: Autonomic disturbances following tibial nerve palsy is very common.

Surgical treatment may consists of any of the following:
• Posterior transfer of tibialis anterior along with extensor hallucies longus to the first metatarsal to prevent its drop
• Transfer of evertor posteriorly with arthrodesis of subtalar and transverse tarsal joint
• Triple arthrodesis.

Postoperative treatment is given along the same line as that for common peroneal nerve palsy.

FACIAL NERVE PALSY

Causes

Supranuclear Lesion

Supranuclear lesion involving the corticospinal fibers concerning voluntary facial movements. Here the lower part of the face is involved whereas the upper part is relatively spared. The facial palsy in this case is upper motor neuron type of facial palsy.

Supranuclear lesion involving the fibers concerned in emotional movement of the face, e.g. there is a frontal lobe tumor or mimic paralysis.

Nuclear and Infranuclear Lesions

Here the upper part of face is also involved and the paralysis is lower motor neuron type.
• Pontine lesions: Here the facial nerve palsy is associated with V and VI nerve palsy also. Therefore there is paralysis of lateral rectus, conjugate ocular deviation to the same side and paralysis

of ipsilateral jaw muscles. These lesions are tumors, syringo-myelia, vascular lesions, poliomyelitis and multiple sclerosis.

- Within the posterior fossa (between the pons and internal acoustic meatus): Here the facial nerve palsy is associated with the VIII nerve involvement and nervous intermedius. Therefore it is associated with deafness and loss of taste in the anterior 2/3rd of the tongue. These lesions are acoustic neuroma and cerebellar pontine angle tumors.
- Within temporal bone: Within the facial canal, the facial nerve palsy occurs because of the following reasons:
  1. Skull fractures
  2. Infections in the middle ear and mastoid, i.e. Otitis media.
  3. Spread of infection to the facial canal
  4. Surgical operations on the ear
  5. Herpes zoster infection
  6. Mumps
  7. Inflammations of the facial nerve within the stylomastoid foramen.

Delayed facial nerve palsy developing within 1 to 2 weeks after a closed head injury could be due to conduction block of the facial nerve in the facial canal just proximal to the stylomastoid foramen and carries a prognosis which is bad than the Bell's palsy.

- After emerging from the skull the facial nerve may be involved in the inflammation from suppurating glands behind the angle of the jaw or be compressed by tumors or other lesions of the parotid gland.
- Primary degeneration or disorder of the function of facial nerve.

BELL'S PALSY

Bell's palsy is a facial paralysis of acute onset presumed to be due to non-suppurative inflammation of unknown etiology of the facial nerve within its canal above the stylomastoid foramen.

Causes

- History of exposure of the ear to extreme cold
- Water retention in pregnancy
- Infection of the ear
- Herpes zoster infection
- Upper respiratory tract infection
- Idiopathic.

All the above causes facial nerve lesion which begins as neurapraxic type.

Incidence

It occurs any time from infancy to old age. However it is more seen among younger population and males are more affected than females.

Signs and Symptoms

Sensory

There is no sensory loss as the sensory branches arises from proximal part of the facial nerve whereas Bell's palsy involves the distal area of the nerve.

Motors

The muscles that are paralyzed are frontalis, corrugator supercili, orbicularis oculi, nasalis, levator labi superioris and inferioris, risorius, buccinator, depressor labi orbicularis oris and mentalis.

The facial nerve palsy is of sudden onset. The lesions is usually unilateral and rarely bilateral. Frequently pain is at the onset in the ear, mastoid region, angle of the jaw or patient may have temporal headache which can be considered as a warning signal.

A complete interruption of the facial nerve at the stylomastoid foramen results in paralysis of all muscles of expression. Upper and lower facial muscles are usually equally affected and voluntary, emotional and associated movements are involved.

The following features may be seen in Bell's palsy (Figs 6.13A to C, Plate 5)
- Drooping of the corner of the mouth
- Creases and skin fold of the face becomes smoothened
- There will be drooping of the eyebrows and wrinkles of the brow are smoothened out
- Forehead is without furrowing
- Owing to the paralysis of the orbicularis oculi, the palpebral fissures is wider on the affected side and closure of the eye is impossible.

When the patient attempts to close his eyes his eyeball will move upward and slightly inward this is called as *Bell's phenomenon.*

Eversion of the lower eyelid called as Ectoprism impairs absorption of tears which tend to overflow the lower eyelid.

- Retraction of mouth and pursing of the lip is not possible
- Paralysis of buccinator leads to accumulation of food between the teeth and the cheek, there will also be dribbling of saliva from the corner of the mouth.
- Patient complains of heaviness or numbness of the face
- Taste is intact
- Distortion of the mouth causes the tongue to deviate to the sound side when protruded thus giving false impression of the hypoglossal lesion.

When the inflammation process extends upwards to involve the nerve above the point at which chorda tympani leaves it all the above symptoms occurs including the following:

- Loss of taste sensation in the anterior two third of the tongue
- If the nerve to stapedius is involved then hyperacusis develop
- If the geniculate ganglion or the motor nerve proximal to it is involved then lacrimation may be reduced. Infact lesion at this point will also involve the VIII cranial nerve
- When the return of the motor function begins the smoothened nasolabial fold starts deepening.
- Attempts to move one group of facial muscles results in contraction of all of them. This is called as associated movements or synkinesis.
- Spasm of facial muscles develop and persist indefinitely by getting initiated with any facial movement. This is called as hemifacial spasm.
- Sometimes there may be anomalous regeneration of the facial nerve which results in any of the event as under:
  1. If the fibers originally connected with the orbicularis oculi become connected with the orbicularis oris, closure of the lid may cause a retraction of the corner of the mouth.
  2. If the visceromotor fibers originally innervating the salivary glands later come to innervate the lacrimal glands, anomalous tearing which is also called as crocodile tears may occur whenever the patient salivates.

Investigations

Strength duration curve, electromyography and nerve conduction studies.

Prognosis

More than 50 percent of the patient may recover although.

MANAGEMENT FOR BELL'S PALSY

1. *Resolving the Inflammation*: If the patient comes immediately following the onset of paralysis, then he may be treated with either SWD or IR to increase the circulation in the stylomastoid foramen so that the inflammation can be resolved. If the paralysis is only due to compression or neurapraxia then the patient will show a miraculous recovery once the inflammation is resolved and compression on the nerve is relieve. Such heat modalities can be tried for a period of one week to ten days.

2. *Maintenance of muscle properties*: This can be achieved with Interrupted galvanic stimulation to the paralyzed muscles.

3. *Facial Massage*: Massage is essential to maintain the circulation to the face as well as to keep the face supple. The direction of the manipulation used should be in upward direction and not downward direction as downward movements tend to stretch the paralyzed muscles more and can have deleterious effect.

4. *Taping or Splinting*: These methods are used to decrease the facial asymmetry noticed in Bell's Palsy

5. *Eye care*: The patient may be instructed to wear protective goggles to prevent entry of foreign bodies into his eyes.

6. *Continuous monitoring*: The patient recovery status should be reviewed consistently. SDC is helpful in knowing the prognosis of the patient.

7. *Faradic Reeducation*: Only if patient can tolerate sensory stimulus of faradic current to the face, faradic reeducation is given. Other means of reeducating the movement is by using PNF techniques, visual feedback exercises etc.

8. *Visual Feedback exercises*: The patient may be asked to do facial exercises in front of the mirror, so that he gets a visual feedback and can perform the exercises more efficiently.

9. *Strengthening exercises:* Once the facial muscles reach grade 3 or fair then resistance can be given to muscle action to further strengthen them.

SELF-ASSESSING QUESTIONS

- Draw brachial plexus and write about brachial plexus injury.
- Describe the clinical features and management of radial, ulnar and median nerve palsy.
- Describe the management of common peroneal nerve palsy.
- Essay on Bell's palsy. What is Bell's phenomenon?
- Difference between upper motor neuron and lower motor neuron type of facial palsy.
- Splints used in various nerve palsy.

7

Physiotherapy in Polyneuropathy

The term polyneuropathy and polyneuritis are usually used as synonyms. However, pathologically speaking polyneuropathy refers to those conditions where there is primary degeneration in the nerve parenchyma which is often triggered by toxins metabolic or vascular causes; whereas polyneuritis refers to inflammation of the connective tissues in the peripheral nerves due to toxins, allergens, and infective conditions.

CLASSIFICATION

Polyneuropathy are broadly classified in two major categories, based upon whether they primarily involve the axon or myelin sheath, as demyelination, axonopathy and wallerian degeneration.

Demyelination means there is abnormality in the myelin covering that causes a decrease in nerve conduction. These can be localized or generalized. The recovery is rapid and complete.

Axonopathy or axonal degeneration means damage to the axon due to metabolic, toxic, infective or traumatic causes. Nerve conduction studies show a decrease in amplitude of the resulting motor unit action potential.

In wallerian degeneration there is demyelination along with axonal disorganization causing chromatolysis of soma. Recovery is slow and incomplete.

ASSESSMENT

Apart from demographic data, complaints and history, the following assessment are essential in polyneuropathy.

Observation

The attitude of limbs, wasting of the muscles, deformity and tropic changes involving the skin, should be observed. In case the patient is on a ventilatory assistance, as in cases of acute cases of Guillaian

Barré syndrome, the setting of the ventilator, vital parameter displayed on the pulse oximeter, etc. should be recorded.

Examination

Cranial Nerve Testing

The cranial nerve are bound to be affected in some types of poly-neuropathy and thus determines the severity and prognosis of the disease.

Sensory Examination

May be grossly affected in cases of some predominant sensory neuropathy like diabetic neuropathy, but usually patient may give complain of abnormal sensation like tingling numbness, paresthesia, walking on cotton, etc.

ROM Testing: Both active a passive ROM should be tested, tightness or contracture should be identified.

Manual Muscle Testing (MMT)

Manual muscle testing is the most important examination procedure to be carried. The muscle should be graded from 1 to 5. Individual muscle testing is a must as it gives an idea about the extent and distribution of weakness thus giving an indication about the various nerves involved.

Reflexes

Deep tendon and superficial reflexes should be checked. The response of these reflexes do not directly correspond to the degree of muscle weakness. Superficial reflexes may or may not be involved based on the nerve affected.

Endurance test should be performed for certain common activity to find the degree of fatiguability of the muscle.

Test for autonomous dysfunction: The integrity of autonomous fibers in the nerve can be tested by Ninhydrin test and Galvanic skin resistance test (For details refer Chapter 1).

Functional assessment: The patient should be assessed for all the activities of daily living to find the level of independency of the patient. It is noted that based on the distribution of the weakness the patient may have difficulty in carrying various functions like in cases of GBS, where the weakness is more marked in proximal parts of the body, the patient may exhibit difficulty or inability in performing all the weight bearing activities.

Investigation

Electrophysiological studies like electromyography, nerv conduction velocity studies, F latency, H reflexes give adequate clu that help in the diagnostic procedure of the case. Routine blood tes biochemical test to find protein concentration in the cerebrospin. fluid are some of the common investigation done.

Although there are various types of polyneuropathy, but the mo commonest ones treated by physiotherapist are GBS, diabet neuropathy and alcoholic neuropathy hence only these three type of neuropathies are discussed in this chapter.

GUILLAIN-BARRÉ-STROHL (GBS) SYNDROME

Synonyms

AIDP (acute idiopathic demyelinating polyneuropathy), AIP (acute infective polyneuropathy, LGBSS (Landry-Guillain-Barré-Strohl syndrome), AIP (acute idiopathic polyneuropathy).

GBS is defined as acute or subacute symmetrical predominantly motor neuropathy involving more than one peripheral nerves, frequently it may involve the facial and other cranial nerve, doesn't have any known etiology, reaches a peak of disability by 4 weeks, has a monophasic course and usually ends up with recovery.

Predisposing Factor

Although there is no definite etiology of GBS there are certain factors which have been found to predispose to the occurrence of GBS.

Age

Common between 15 to 25 years of age.

Sex

Common in females.

Infection

Viral in the form of Epstein Barr virus, bacterial in the form of mycoplasma pneumonia.

Vaccination

Rabies, typhoid, tetanus, or influenza vaccination may precipitate the attack of GBS.

Surgery

After 4 to 5 weeks of major surgery patient may show signs of GBS which can be attributed to the following reasons:
- release of neural antigen that provokes autoimmune response
- due to surgical stress
- because of blood transfusion.

Drugs

Prolonged use of antidepressant drugs like zimelidine or gold therapy which are neurotoxins are found to cause GBS.

Autoimmune

Due to the presence of an antigen CD +ve T cells.

Idiopathic

Without any known causes.

Clinical Features

- The onset of GBS is acute or subacute.
- Progression: The motor paralysis spreads usually within 30 minutes to four weeks time. It may take on an average of 4 to 5 days for the weakness to reach its peak. Once the weakness reaches its peak it remains at a plateau or it maintains a plateau for 15 to 20 days following which the patient recovers for 4 to 6 months. In rare case the recovery may extend up to 2 years also.
- Motor: Weakness of the muscle which is of LMN type is seen with involvement of more than one limbs. The weakness is usually symmetrical on both sides. The proximal parts are more involved than the distal parts although the disease may start from distal parts. Weakness of the facial and other cranial nerves may cause dysphagia, diplopia and respiratory failure. According to Cooper and his co-worker the weakness of the shoulder elevators and neck flexors are in parallel to the involvement of diaphragm and respiratory failure. Weakness of the trunk and extremities

causes incoordinated jerky movements which is very obvious during gait.

- Sensory: Symptoms range from mild pain to paresthesia. Total loss of sensation is usually not seen. The alteration in sensation is due to ongoing process of degeneration which causes spontaneous discharge by the small myelinated sensory fibers.
- Areflexia: This occurs in GBS and does not necessarily corresponds to weakness. It is usually due to asynchronization in the firing by the motor axon. Synchronization of the discharge along the reflex arc is very essential to elicit a monosynaptic reflex. In GBS as there is demyelination it causes lack of synchronization in the firing by the motor axon.
- Myalgia or muscular pain occurs because of release of a substance called cytokinin by the macrophages at the inflammatory foci of the nerve terminal. This substance causes damage to the muscles thereby irritating the nerve endings in the muscles.
- Sphincter disturbance: The patient may have retention or overflow incontinence based upon the involvement of sympathetic or parasympathetic fibers supplying the urinary bladder.
- Autonomic disturbance: Orthostatic hypotension is common in the patient with GBS due to the lack of sympathetic mediated vascular response that causes peripheral pooling of blood. Sweating may be totally lost or profuse.

Investigation

The albumin level in the CSF is increased during the course of muscular weakness and it may remain increased even for 4 weeks after the muscular weakness has reached the plateau. Eventually it reaches to the baseline.

Electrophysiology shows an neurogenic type of presentation with an increase in the amplitude, increase in the duration of the motor unit potential with polyphasia. With increased resistance the muscles exhibit delayed and incomplete interference pattern.

Diagnostic Criteria

Acute onset, symmetrical involvement, predominantly proximal weakness, more than one limb involved, areflexia, orthostatic hypotension and almost complete recovery are some of the important diagnostic criteria to detect GBS.

Medical Management

- Plasmapheresis
- Steroid therapy
- Injection of IgG (Immunoglobulin-G)

PT Management

Chest Physiotherapy

In the initial stages if the patient is on respiratory assistance then the patient has to be regularly seen by the therapist. The aims of the management in this stage consists of the following:

- Maintain clear airways and to prevent respiratory complication
- Continuous change of position to drain out secretion and also to facilitate proper air entry to all the lobes of the lung.
- Periodic suctioning in a strictly hygienic manner.
- Percussion, shaking, manual mobilization with the help of ambubag may be necessary to loosen out the secretion.
- Nebulization in case of any respiratory infection.

However if the patient is not on ventilator then chest physiotherapy technique like breathing exercise, postural drainage, external tracheal stimulation may be given to maintain good bronchial hygiene.

Maintenance of Range of Motion at All Joints

The range of motion can be maintained by passive range of motion exercises. Slow gradual stretching especially of the biarticular muscles is very essential to prevent tightness of these soft tissue structure. Passive movements should be given at least three times in a day involving all the movements at all the joints. Each movements should be repeated at least five times during each sitting.

Support to the Limbs

Static splints are given to prevent contracture as well as to immobilize the part to prevent any unwanted damage to the muscles or joints. Splints are commonly used for the foot and hand to maintain it in neutral position. Even pillows may be used to support various body parts.

Pain relief

Patient with GBS in the acute stage suffer from pain and paresthesia which may interfere with the rehabilitation process hence to give patient relief from these altered sensation TENS may be used.

Maintenance of Muscle Properties

Muscles begin to atrophy very rapidly in these condition hence *Functional Electrical Stimulation* may be used to maintain the muscle property. Even stimulation with interrupted direct current to the functionally important muscles may be given to maintain their properties.

Prevention and Treatment of Pressure Sores

Pressure sore can be prevented by constantly changing the posture, gentle massage of the pressure prone areas, by keeping the skin dry and soft as well as by giving mattress which help in more even distribution of the weight. In case pressure sores do develop then measures like ice cube massage around the wound, UVR radiation, LASER, etc. radiation etc. may be used to treat the sore.

Prevention of Postural Hypotension

Postural hypotension is very common in this case due to the combine effect of severe hypotonicity and supine position. This can be prevented by stimulation of the vascular reflex by getting the patient into an erect position very gradually using a tilt table and by using elastocrepe bandage.

Psychological Support

The patient motivation must be kept high. He should be told about the treatment and its significance which will be helpful in improving the out come of the rehabilitation.

Once the patient comes out of the acute stage then the physiotherapy treatment can become more vigorous. The main aim of the treatment in this stage involves:
- Strengthening of the weak muscles
- Functional reeducation
- Gait training
- Respiratory and cardiovascular conditioning

Strengthening

IG stimulation can be continued till the patient is able to generate contraction of the muscles voluntary but is unable to perform any movement (grade 1). Once the patient reaches grade 1 then he can be given Faradic reeduction by using short surge faradic current, this can be continued till he is able to perform the action in a gravity eliminated position. To improve the grade from 2 to grade 3, patient may be exercised actively by using reeducation board or smooth exercise table, suspension therapy, and other form of active assisted exercise. Once the patient reaches grade 3 then resisted exercises can be given using manual resistance, springs, pulleys, weights, hydrotherapy, etc. It should be remembered that it is preferable to give this resisted exercises in the pattern of functional significance.

Functional Training

It is essential to incorporate the improvement in the muscle strength into various activities of daily living. For certain patient with a very gradual improvement, functional electrical stimulation or orthosis may be used to perform a functional task.

Gait Training

Gait training is initiated in the parallel bar and then progressed to walking unsupported on an even surface within the clinic. Once the patient walks quite comfortable and confidently on even floor, then the challenge can be increased by making the patient walk on uneven surface.

Sensory deficit is not marked in GBS patient, hence sensory reeducation may not be always given.

Most of the patient with GBS improve to a remarkable extent within the initial two years of time. The ultimate improvement is strictly based on the number of nerves involved and the severity of their involvement.

DIABETIC NEUROPATHY

About 15 percent of the patient with diabetes develop neuropathy complication. Although not all will produce signs and symptoms. There are different types of diabetic neuropathy which are as follows.

Diabetic Mononeuropathy

Only one or two nerves are involved. Most common cranial nerves involved are third cranial nerves which causes weakness of the extraocular muscles giving rise to diabetic ophthalmoplegia. The other cranial nerves that can be frequently involved is sixth cranial nerve. The peripheral nerves are not usually involved. Very rarely there is involvement of either sciatic or femoral nerve. The exact mechanism of neurogenic involvement is not known. However, it may be due to involvement of the vascular supply to the nerves causing infarction.

Multiple Mononeuropathy

This can be further divided into two types:
- Rapidly evolving painful asymmetrical predominantly sensory neuropathy.
- Rapidly evolving painless asymmetrical predominantly motor neuropathy.

The first variety is very common in older age group with mild to moderate neuropathy. The patients mainly has pain at the back which may be radiating to the hip and even down to the thigh. The pain is deep and aching in character and usually aggravates at night. Deep tendon jerks may be involved at the knee mainly due to involvement of the sensory pathway of the reflex arc. Motor symptoms are very rare and are usually confined to hip and thigh musculature.

Unlike the above the second variety is predominantly motor neuropathy causing gross weakness and wasting of the proximal muscles at the hip, the thigh, and even involving the scapula and the shoulder. Sensory symptoms are very rare and if present may manifest as mild pain in the involved area. Reflexes may be reduced because of the weakness of the muscles.

Thoracoabdominal Neuropathy

In this type of neuropathy the patient has pain along one or two segments of the thoracic spine. The pain may radiate horizontally from the back to involve the abdominal area. EMG studies have shown fibrillation potentials of the back muscles and abdominal muscles confirming the involvement of spinal nerve roots.

The above type of neuropathies generally have a good prognosis and faster recovery.

Distal Symmetric Neuropathy

Most common type seen in diabetic patient. Usually begins with mild sensory symptoms of pain or paresthesia which gradually spreads. The sensory symptoms in the form of pain or paresthesia usually worsens at night and are usually confined to the distal most part of the extremities. Usually the altered sensation are present in the foot and distal leg area and very rarely may also involve the hand and wrist. This type of involvement of both the upper and lower limb has been termed as "glove and stocking" appearance.

In the later stages the patient may have involvement of the joints causing arthropathy and may eventually cause charcot joints. Ankle jerks are usually affected due to involvement of the sensory fibers of reflex pathway.

Autonomic Neuropathy

Autonomic disturbances like pupillary and lacrimal dysfunction may be noted in diabetic patients. There may be either increase or decrease of sweating. The most common autonomic disturbance seen in diabetic patient is postural hypotension which occur due to peripheral pooling of blood. The exact cause of autonomic involvement is not properly understood. However the following three mechanism have been put forth.
- Accumulation of vacuoles and granules in sympathetic ganglia
- Demyelination of the nerve fibers
- Loss of cell in the intermediate lateral column in the spinal cord.

Note Decrease tone of the GIT bowel causes nocturnal diarrhea. The patient may have reduced tone of the bladder.

Investigation

Blood sugar level, urine sugar level and EMG are the common investigation which help in the diagnosis of this condition.

Medical Management

Insulin and aldostatin are commonly used.

Physiotherapy management

Unlike GBS, in diabetic neuropathy the sensory symptoms are more dominating hence the management also differs accordingly.

Relief of pain or paresthesia: As the patient with diabetes have pain or paresthesia due to the ongoing process of degeneration of the sensory fibres. This can be alleviated because of IFT or TENS which is given along the course of the painful area.

Care of anesthetic hand and foot: The area involved should be carefully inspected at a regular interval of time to look out for any minor cuts or aberrations and should take immediate measures to control it otherwise ignoring this minor wound may cause major ulceration in future.

- The affected part should be kept quite clean and after every washed it should be dabbed properly with a towel as wet skins are prone to develop infections.
- In case of dry weather pliability of the skin should be maintained by use of moisturizing cream or oil because dryness will precipitate a break in the skin which may encourage all forms of infection.
- The person should be instructed to use protective wears in the form of hand gloves, shoes both in and out side the house.
- The footwear should be made of microcellular material so that any form of soreness of the foot due to pressure within the shoe may be prevented.
- Certain house hold adaptations are essential especially of the utensils to avoid any cut or burns to the hand and feet. Thus the utensil should be properly insulated with proper handle to avoid any casualty.

Prevention of postural hypotension: Abdominal binders and elastic stockings for lower limbs are given to prevent any peripheral pooling of blood thus preventing postural hypotension. The patient may be gradually got into an erect posture by using a tilt table. In case of muscle weakness the menagement is similar to GBS.

Alcoholic Neuropathy

Synonyms: Nutritional or alcoholic neuropathy, beriberi or vitamin B deficiency syndrome.

The neurological manifestation which is seen is mainly due to vitamin B_{12} deficiency is called as beriberi which can affect any organs in the body but the frequently involved organs are the heart and peripheral nerves. Dr. Shattuck in 1928 found out that an excellent relationship between alcoholism and neurological manifestation of alcoholism is due to lack of vitamin B_{12}. He has provided enough evidence to prove that alcoholism doesn't produce direct toxic effect on the nerves and the neuropathy that is seen is mainly because of the inability of the alcoholics to assimilate the food that is rich in vitamin B_{12}.

Pathology

There is gross degeneration of the axon as well as the myelin sheath. Segmental demyelination may also be seen but the proportion of nerve fibers involved is very less. In extreme cases the anterior and posterior roots of the spinal nerves may also be involved. The vagus and the phrenic nerve may be involved in rare cases.

Signs and Symptoms

* *Pain and paresthesia*: This is felt by the patient at the feet or distal leg and sometimes even in the hand. The sensation may range from dull ache to severe stabbing sensation that is felt along the course of the peripheral nerve. The patient may at times have altered sensations of extreme cold and burning feet syndrome. This is also called Dyesthesia.

* *Hyperpathia*: This is a disorder of increased sensitivity in which even the mild touch sensation is wrongly interpreted and is perceived as severe painful sensation.

* *Motor symptoms:* These are not specific but are disproportionate and may vary From cases to cases. Some patients may have proximal muscles more involved than distal. Sometimes the distal muscles are more involved than the proximal. Sometimes the weakness is evenly distributed. Weakness of the muscles lead to muscular imbalance which in turn leads to contractures and deformity. Tenderness of the muscles is often a common complain which can be checked by squeezing the calf muscles.

* *Reflexes:* They are either absent or depressed and may be due to the involvement of the sensory or motor fibers.

- *Autonomic dysfunction:* Patient experiences excessive sweating at the palm and the sole. Orthostatic hypotension may be experienced by the patient in case of involvement of sympathetic fibers. Involvement of the vagus nerve causes dysphasia and hoarseness of the voice.

- *Respiratory complication:* Involvement of the phrenic nerve causes diaphragmatic dysfunction and respiratory problems.

Investigation

CSF examination: Normal electrophysiologic studies shows decreased nerve conduction velocity. EMG studies show neurogenic signs with fibrillation potential.

Management

Modification of dietary habit: The patient should be asked to consume food which is rich in vitamin B.

Aspirin may be used to control pain and paresthesia.

PT management is same as that of GBS.

SELF-ASSESSING QUESTIONS

- Discuss assessment of sensory motor neuropathies.
- Discuss the problem of patient with neuropathies.
- Describe the management of patient with sensory motor neuropathy.
- Care of anesthetic hand and foot.
- Write a note on GBS.
- Short notes on diabetic neuropathy.
- Short notes on alcoholic neuropathy.
- What is the cause of myalgia in GBS.

8

Physiotherapy in Muscular Dystrophy

Although there are various types of muscular dystrophy that have been found out over the years but there are only few which are frequently met by a therapist. This chapter thus will focus on the clinical aspect of such dystrophies along with giving a treatment outline towards the management of muscular dystrophy in general.

DUCHENNE MUSCULAR DYSTROPHY (DMD)

Duchenne dystrophy is not only the most common and also the most severe types of muscular dystrophy.

Incidence

This dystrophy is seen in 1 out of 3,000 to 4,000 male babies born. As the disease is linked it is noticed only in males. The female carrier transmits the disease through genes to the male child. In majority of the female carrier there is no apparent signs or symptoms.

Clinical Presentation

The disease may not show ány indication during the early infancy although in some of the child walking may not be attained even at eighteen months of age.

Onset

The disease is usually noticed at about three years of age. It has a subacute type of onset. The parents may notice a very slow clumpsy walking in their child with frequent falls. Climbing upstairs becomes a very laborious work and cannot be attained without any support.

Progression

Gradually the child develops a lordotic posture due to gross weakness of the abdominal muscles. Getting up from squatting is impossible without support and the child adopts the typical Gower's sign which consists of a typical getting up manner by the child using support of various parts in the lower limb. It appears as though he is climbing up into standing using support of his lower limb. He develops waddling gait and is no longer able to jump or run around like any other kids of his age. Walking becomes progressively difficult. For some period the child may continue to be ambulant with the help of orthosis, but eventually by around 8 to 12 years he is confined to bed and mobility can be achieved only with the help of wheelchair.

Weakness

The muscular weakness will be typically of a lower motor neuron type. The muscles which commonly develop progressive weakness are plantar flexors, evertors, quadriceps, gluteus muscles, long extensors of the hand, biceps, triceps, deltoid, pectoralis, latissimus dorsi and some shoulder girdle muscles.

Hypertrophy

In contrast to other lower motor neuron type of disorder where there is wasting, DMD child will show hypertrophy of certain muscles like plantar flexors, quadriceps, deltoid, temporalis, hip extensors and even pectoralis. This hypertrophies is called as *Pseudohypertrophy* as it is caused due to abnormal deposition of fatty tissue and fibrous tissue in the muscle mass.

Reflexes

The superficial reflexes are lost and eventually even the deep tendon jerks are lost.

Contracture and Deformity

The muscular imbalance produced makes the limb and trunk prone for developing contractures and deformity. Hip deformity due to TFL contractures, knee flexion deformity, ankle plantar flexion deformity, lordosis, scoliosis, etc. are noticed.

Functional Independency

The functional capacity of the child keeps deteriorating day by day and eventually the child will be totally dependent for dressing, bathing, toileting and even rolling in bed at night.

Respiratory Insufficiency

Although diaphragm is the only muscles which is never involved in DMD, respiratory complication are inevitable in this condition mainly because of the total inactivity. The child frequently gets respiratory infection due to lack of mobility and adequate chest expansion. Death is usually due to respiratory complication.

Intelligence

Usually the mean IQ of these children is around 75 to 80 percent. However it does not deteriorate with age.

GIT Abnormalities

Due to immobility the child may have constipation, vomiting due to pressure of superior mesenteric vessels on the third part of duodenum may be noted.

Obesity

Due to total inactivity and compensatory over eating the child may put on too much of weight if not guided properly.

Emotional Disturbances

The constant deterioration of the child comes as a shock to the family member who generally needs sometime to understand the situation completely and cope up with it. Needless to say, both the child and the parents are depressed looking at the helpless situation.

Investigative Findings

- The CPK level is very high
- EMG shows typical myogenic pictures with small amplitude, small duration polyphasic potential. The interference pattern is early. Sometimes lateron during the course of the disease there may be presence of fasciculation potentials.
- The muscle biopsy will show extensive variation in the size of the fibers with increased infiltration of fatty tissues and fibrous tissues.

PT Management

The management of dystrophy is a team approach and none of the team member can ever claim superior influence then his counterpart because it requires interdisciplinary approach the stage of influence by various rehabilitation professional may be different.

The physiotherapist role in a child with muscular dystrophy consists of the following:

Parental Counseling

Unlike parents of children with neurological problems such as CP, polio, etc. the parents of a child with dystrophy tends to develop a psychological state which is different from a stage of shock. They have seen a child born normal, attaining a normal milesstone, leading a absolutely normal life like any other kid and then gradually deteriorating. They find it difficult of accept this fact and always tend to think Is there some way the whole process can be stopped if not completely reversed? The therapist needs to speak to the parents in a very clever manner without totally putting the parents off guard suddenly. The fact need to be spoken to so that the parents doesn't get fooled by believing that their child will become absolutely normal some day. Infact only if they know the fact better will they be able to contribute better in the treatment process.

Also since as in most of the DMD the mothers and the sisters of the child are carriers they need to take counseling from a geneticist and gynecologist before trying to conceive again. In developing countries like our where people from rural areas are mostly illiterate and uncivilized the usual tendency for them to think is that since one child is having this disability probably the other child born will lead a normal life and thus will be taking a great risk. Thus they need to be counselled in a polite and correct ways regarding this probability.

Exercises

The patient should be encouraged to lead active life as long as possible. Activities of daily living by itself can strengthen and maintain flexibility of various muscles in the functional range. Mild strengthening techniques especially using PNF techniques like Repeated contraction can prove to be beneficial. The therapist should avoid giving vigorous strengthening exercises as they may aggravated damage to the muscles and thus may prove to be more harmful than beneficial. Of course the functional capacity of the child will decline consistently but one should aim at prolonging the independence capacity of the child. In addition to trying and maintaining the muscle strength and property as long as possible, the therapist should also give mobility exercises to the child. These mobility exercises taught should be simple and something that the child can do actively in the house without having to depend on someone else assistance. Parents of the child may also be taught these exercises so that they can assist the child especially in the later stages. Suspension and modification in the therapeutic exercises should be determined by periodic rechecks at least once every three months.

Preventing Contractures

Contractures sets in very early and are quite severe which could be due to direct involvement of the muscle itself. The two joint muscles of the body like the gastrocnemius, tensor fascia lata, rectus femoris and hamstring in the lower limb are very prone to develop tightness and contractures. In the upper extremity, the forearm pronators, wrist flexors, finger flexors are often tight. Simple stretching techniques for these muscles may be taught to the parents so that these exercises can be done at home. Advises like lying prone for some time everyday will prevent hip flexion deformity. This can be done while watching TV, while playing some games, etc. Stretching should be done gently but up to maximum range possible so that walking can be retained as long as possible. After sometimes splinting may become necessary especially to maintain knee extension, ankle dorsiflexion. But the splint should be made of light polypropylene type of material so that it can be used as functional splint also.

Deformities of the lower limb can cause multiple secondary problems like for instance asymmetric muscle tightness of an iliotibial band causes scoliosis at the spine, pelvic tilt, subluxation of the hip, etc. The collapsing spine needs proper support. Braces to maintain extension of the spine becomes necessary to prevent undue strain on the vertebral column which can otherwise cause mechanical pain that will only add on to the discomfort to the patient.

Home Adaptation

Modification in the house for easy accessibility and functional independence of the patient can be best brought about by contributions from therapist, social workers and local housing authority. The pathways, width of the doorway, provision of ramps or lift, support bars in the toilet, accessibility of the patient into various rooms, should be considered in the modification agenda.

The height of the bed, chair and toilet are critical for independence. Moreover at one stage the parents or attainder may have to transfer the child by lifting hence the height of various furniture is very essential. The mattresses should be firm and resilient so that bed activities and transfer of the patient becomes easier. In later stages providing an alarm bell near to the cot of the child will make night care much more easier.

Schooling

In the initial stages when the child is ambulant local schools can manage but as the child's weakness becomes quite increase such that it interferes with his walking then at that stage special schools may be necessary. Sending the child with gross muscular weakness to ordinary schools will definitely set a complexity in him which may interfere with his mind set preventing him from concentrating on his education. Moreover normal schools are not accessible for wheelchair bound people thereby locomotion of the child becomes difficult.

Recreational Activities

As the child is absolutely normal mentally he is well aware of his deteriorating situation but cannot resists the temptation of getting involved in various sports despite experiencing some sense of difficulty. Hence the parents should wisely advice the child against getting involved in various contact sports that may cause further injuries. But some kind of recreational activity should be given which won't be physically demanding like playing carom, chess, watching television, bird watching, fishing, etc. The situation is quite pitiful because unlike a mentally retarded child, a child with muscular dystrophy has all the desire to enjoy games of a physically normal child but is forced to abstain from these.

Encouraging Functional Independency

The usual age at which walking becomes impossible varies between 8 to 12. The therapist should encourage walking as long as possible because it is one of the ways of exercising the muscles of the lower extremities. Also walking keeps the spine in extension as well as prevents any contractures and deformity. But too much of exertion should be discouraged at each stages of this condition. In the initial stages the child walks without any calliperization but eventually he will need some light weighted orthosis to continue walking. As the condition is progressive the functional independency of the child keeps deteriorating. It is not in our capacity to prevent this deterioration but one should make all possible attempt to slow down this process of deterioration and try to keep the child active as long as possible.

Lifting Techniques and Transfer

By the time a child becomes totally non-ambulant, he is already quite grown up and may even become heavy due to lack of mobility hence the parents, teacher and other attainders of the child are taught correct lifting techniques like use of belt, so that they don't strain themselves. The child may be taught how to roll over in the bed, use of sliding boards etc. for transfer. However the child should be encouraged to carry out all his activities on his own as long as possible.

Wheel chair Management

Once the child no longer is able to walk even with orthosis then it is more wiser to advise him to use the wheelchair. The wheel chair should be used only as a mode of transfer because more time the child spends on the wheelchair more is the chances for him to develop contractures and deformity. Initially the child may be able to manage maneuvering the wheelchair with his hand but as the weakness progresses further involving the upper limb musculature then a motorized wheel chair becomes necessary. However in Indian condition managing with a wheelchair becomes difficult due to horrible road conditions, inadequate space in the house, etc. The wheelchair should be of appropriate size for the child so that sitting posture of the child is good with 90 degree angulation at the knee, foot support should be good, the back support should be such that the child doesn't stoop or side bend to any one side. When the muscle power becomes poor and the child is unable to maintain his position in the wheelchair, lateral support or strapping may be added.

Secondary Complication that Needs to be Prevented

Due to progressive muscular weakness and immobility, the child should be prevented from developing the following secondary complication, which will only increase the discomfort of the patient.

Spinal Deformity

Muscular imbalance to the trunk coupled with abnormal sitting posture can cause spinal deformities like scoliosis and kyphosis. Hence the spine of the child should be regularly inspected for spinal deformity. Various stretching procedures may be carried out to prevent opposite group of muscles from going into contractures. Spinal braces with proper padding may be given to prevent the spinal deformities from aggravating.

Obesity

Lack of normal mobility makes the child weight gain. The diet of the child should be strictly the ones rich in protein and carbohydrate without any fat. Eating habit should be properly supervised to prevent the child from becoming a mechanical eater who is being left out with less other options.

Fractures

As the ambulation of the child becomes more and more difficult the chances of the child falling and developing a fracture is more. Moreover due to decreased weight bearing, there is demineralization of the bone which increases the chances of stress fracture. The chances increases especially when the child is walking around with his callipers. This can be prevented if the child is kept under careful observation and not allowing him to walk alone in places where there is lot of obstacle.

SELF-ASSESSING QUESTIONS

Long and Short Essay

- What are the clinical features of DMD?
- What is the PT management of DMD?
- What are the various ways of coping with the problem of a child suffering from DMD?
- Significance of parental counseling and home adaptation for DMD.

Short Answers

- What is dystrophin?
- Investigation for muscular dystrophy.
- EMG finding in DMD.

9

Spinal Cord Diseases

Before one goes into the actual clinical aspect of spinal cord diseases it is necessary to brush through the structures present in the spinal cord and the functions of these structures (Fig. 9.1).

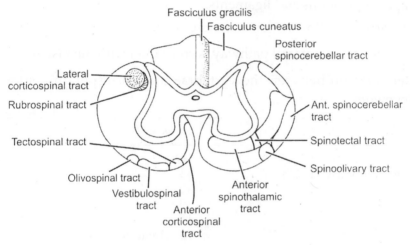

Fig. 9.1: Transverse section of the spinal cord

Descending Tracts

Corticospinal tract: Voluntary movements, controls finer movements of the fingers.

Rubrospinal tracts: Facilitates flexors movements, inhibits extensor muscles.

Vestibulospinal tracts: Facilitates extensors, inhibits flexors.

Reticulospinal tracts: Facilitates or inhibits muscle activity.

Tectospinal tract: Tectal reflex (vision).

Ascending Tracts

Medial leminiscus: Carries joint position sense, tactile localization, 2 point discrimination, vibration and fine touch. It acts at conscious level.

Lateral spinothalamic tract: Lateral spinothalamic tract carries temperature and pain.

Anterior spinothalamic tract: It carries crude touch and pressure sensation.

Spinocerebellar tract: It works at unconscious level and carrier kinesthetic sensation from the muscles, fascia, skin.

Spino-olivary tract: It carries messages to the superficial fascia, capsules, tendons and ligaments.

Spinoreticular: It works on conscious level.

Spinotectal: Spinotectal pathway is concerned with the vision.

Relationship between the vertebrae and corresponding spinal segments.

Vertebrae	Spinal segments
Upper cervical (C1 to C4)	Same
Lower cervical (C4 to C7)	+1
T1-T7	+2
T7-T9	+3
T12	L5
L1	Sacral and coccygeal

CLASSIFICATION OF SPINAL CORD DISEASES

1. *Compressive*
   - Intramedullary tumors
   - Extramedullary tumors
   - Epidural abscess
   - Epidural hemorrhage
   - Cervical spondylosis
   - PID of cervical or lumbar area
   - Traumatic compression of the spinal cord
2. *Vascular*
   - Atriovenous malformation

3. *Inflammatory*
   - Acute transverse myelitis
   - Myelopathy
   - Multiple sclerosis

4. *Infective*
   - Tabes Dorsalis
   - Parasitic and bacterial infections

5. *Developmental*
   - Syringomyelia

6. *Metabolic*
   - Subacute combined degeneration

7. *Congenital*
   - Spina bifida with myelocele or meningomyelocele

8. *Degenerative*
   - Motor neuron disease

9. *Traumatic.*

Disorders of the spinal cord can be either causing quadriplegia or paraplegia. Quadriplegia is a condition in which all the four limbs, trunk and the respiratory muscles are affected. Damage is at cervical part of the spinal column.

Paraplegia is affection of the lower limbs and may not necessarily affect the trunk and respiratory muscles. It is caused due to damage to the thoracic and lumbar level spine.

Spinal cord injury could be complete or incomplete depending on the severity of lesion.

Complete lesions is in which all the sensations and motor fibers below the level of the lesions is lacking. The recovery or prognosis is bad and those lesions are usually seen following a complete transection of spinal cord, extensive vascular insufficiency or severe cord compression.

Incomplete lesions are the one in which some sensory, motor fibers are intact because some visible neural tissues escape the damage at the site of the lesion. This is usually seen following a contusion due to compression by bone fragments or other soft tissues or due to partial damage to the spinal cord. Recovery is variable, may be good or bad. Early return of function is a good prognostic sign.

Affection Pattern

Brown-Séquard Syndrome

This is caused mainly due to stab injuries or other trauma that damages one side of the spinal cord. Due to this there will be loss of pain temperature and crude touch on opposite side whereas loss of tactile localization and two point discrimination, joint position sensation on same side below the level of lesion. Also as the lesion progresses there will be involvement of the motor neuron that leads to weakness, wasting and loss of jerks at the site of lesion due to destruction of anterior horn cell at that level. Involvement of the descending tracts will cause spastic weakness below the level of lesion due to affection of the pyramidal tract. This kind of clinical presentation is called as Brown-Séquard syndrome (Fig. 9.2).

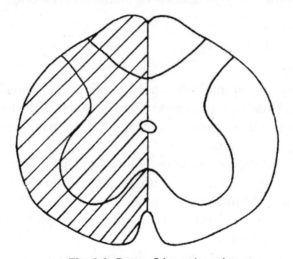

Fig. 9.2: Brown-Séquard syndrome

Anterior Cord Syndrome (Fig. 9.3)

This is caused by blockage or rupture of anterior spinal artery, space occupying lesion or a mass compressing from anterior aspect, hyperflexion injuries of spinal column. As the anterior part of the spinal cord is damaged there is loss of pain, temperature sensation below the level of the lesion. There may be damage of the anterior horn cell at the level of the lesion giving rise to lower motor neuron picture of the muscles supplied by those anterior horn cell of the cord. There may be spastic paraparesis below the level of lesion but the sensation carried by posterior column remains intact.

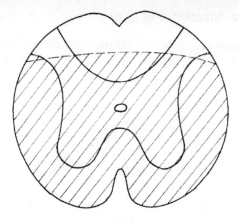

Fig. 9.3: Anterior cord syndrome

Central Cord Syndrome (Fig. 9.4)

Involvement of the central cord of the spinal column causes affection of pain and temperature sensations as these fibers cross near the central column. Therefore there is loss of pain and temperature sensation in the proximal part whereas the sacral part is spared. Perianal sensations, contractions of rectal sphincter and sensation of the saddle area are intact. The toe flexors that are supplied by sacral segments are normal and this presentation is sacral sparing.

The causes of central cord syndrome are syringomyelia, tumors near the central canal, ischemia of the anterior spinal artery, hyperextension injury.

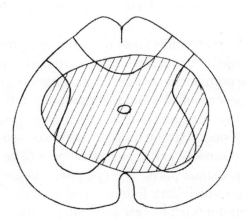

Fig. 9.4: Central cord syndrome

Posterior Column Affection (Fig. 9.5)

As there is damage to posterior column or dorsal column all the sensations carried by this column are absent below the level of lesion. This leads to sensory ataxia and is usually caused by *tabes dorsalis*.

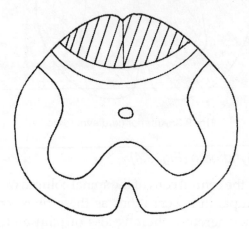

Fig. 9.5: Posterior cord syndrome

Cauda Equina Lesions

Complete lesion of cauda equina is unusual due to larger surface area and large number of nerve roots. Clinical presentation is similar to any nerve injuries which consists of weakness, wasting and loss of reflexes. Complete recovery following a central cord lesion does not always occur due to reasons like:

• Distance between the site of lesion and point of reinnervation is more.
• The regenerating nerve fibers may not follow the previous course.
• Glial and collagen scarring can block the process of regeneration.
• There may be permanent changes in the target organs.
• Process of regeneration slows down gradually and stops.

It is possible to differentiate between Intramedullary and Extramedullary lesion. Extramedullary lesion consists of findings such as the loss of sensory and motor affection will be in the distal and then in the proximal parts. The symptoms begin with severe radicular pain. Intramedullary lesions consists of findings such as the sensory and motor functions are lost in the proximal parts of the body and then the distal parts. Pain is very poorly localized and burning in character. However, the pain and temperature sensation in proximal parts is involved first in intramedullary lesion and distal part is involved first in extramedullary compression for pain and temperature sensation.

Although there are various diseases of the spinal cord, this chapter will focus on only those which are commonly encountered by the physiotherapist in neurological wards and ICU.

SYRINGOMYELIA

It is defined as a chronic progressive degeneration of the spinal cord characterized pathologically by cavitations of the central canal or gray matter of the spinal cord and clinically by brachial amyotrophy and segmental sensory loss of dissociated type.

Etiology

Syringomyelia is usually caused by abnormal formation of posterior fossa and foramen magnum. The conditions that are frequently associated with syringomyelia are:
1. Arnold-Chiari malformation type I
2. Platybasia
3. Dandy-Walker syndrome in which there is cyst in the posterior fossa.

These conditions cause obstruction to the flow of CSF from IV ventricle to the sub acrachnoid space of the spinal cord. There are other less common cases that can give rise to this kind of obstruction. They are:
   a. Dural cyst
   b. Subarachnoiditis
   c. Atlantoaxial fusion
   d. Cerebellar cyst
   e. Basilar artery invagination
   f. Intramedullary tumor of the spinal cord

Pathogenesis

There are several theories that are proposed in order to explain the formation of such syrinx. First theory was proposed by Gardener according to whom obstruction of the foramen Magendie and Luschka blocks the flow of CSF from the fourth ventricle into the subarachnoid space. As a result of which there is formation of a pressure wave within the IV ventricle that exerts a downward push on the fluid into the central matter of the spinal cord.

However this theory was opposed by Ball and Dyan on the basis of fact that there is not always a continuity between the IV ventricle and syrinx. Also they felt that the pressure wave generated within the IV ventricle was not strong enough to push the fluid into the spinal cord. According to them when the outflow of the CSF from the subarachnoid space is blocked and when the situation is complicated by any form of physical exertion like neck mobility the fluid tracks into the spinal cord through Virchow-Robin spaces. This accumulated fluid over a period of time leads to formation of cavity which virtually is independent of central canal but over a period of time coalesces or joins with them.

Classification

1. Syrmgomyelia with obstruction at craniovertebral junction like Arnold-Chiari malformation and any other obstructive lesion.
2. Syringomyelia without obstruction (Idiopathic type).
3. Syringomyelia with other diseases of spinal cord like intra-medullary tumor, compressive myelopathy.
4. Hydromyelia with hydrocephalus (which causes dilatation of the central canal).

Clinical Features

The disease is present since birth but the clinical manifestation occurs during late adolescence and early adult hood (15-20 years).

1. Since the cavities are formed near the central canal the pain and the temperature sensation are the first to be affected. The sensory loss is segmental and dissociated type. However, it may have a "hemicape" distribution in which there is loss of pain and temperature sensation in the lower part of the face like arm, neck and shoulder.
2. There will be weakness and wasting of the muscles supplied by affected segments and it is usually the hand area that is affected. As the cavity expands there may be involvement of the pyramidal pathways leading to spasticity of lower limbs and even sphincter disturbances.
3. Kyphoscoliosis is usually associated with syringomyelia. In case of syringobulbia there will be nystagmus, dysarthria, dysphagia and hoarseness of voice. Less commonly the person may present

with diplopia, trigeminal nerve pain or neuralgia and recurrent hiccups.

Investigations

MRI can usually confirm the diagnosis of syringomyelia.

Treatment

Surgical intervention becomes necessary in most of the cases. The common surgeries performed may be:

Decompression at craniovertebral junction by suboccipital craniotomy or cervical laminectomy. In cases of syrinx in spinal cord a shunting may be done in between the cavity and the subarachnoid space. Shunting also becomes necessary in hydrocephalus with syringomyelia. In cases of intramedullary tumor excisions of the tumor is the choice. Surgical out comes are most often successful especially in the earlier stage of the disease but in some cases it may be of no use.

Physiotherapy Management

1. Care of the anesthetic hand (Refer diabetic neuropathy)
2. Maintenance of range of motion
3. Improve the strength of the muscles
4. Develop coordination if the patient has ataxia due to involvement of the cerebellum as in cases of Arnold Chiari type I malformation.

MOTOR NEURON DISEASE

It is one of the most devastating types of neurological disorder where-in there is a progressive degeneration of motor neurons causing amyotrophy, weakness and corticospinal signs in different combinations.

The cause of motor neuron disease is usually not known however in some cases hereditary factors may be considered.

The motor neuron diseases manifests in different forms like:

1. Amyotrophic lateral sclerosis
2. Progressive muscular atrophy
3. Progressive bulbar palsy
4. Primary lateral sclerosis.

Amyotrophic Lateral Sclerosis

It usually begins at around 40-50 years of age. Men are more affected and about 5 percent cases are predisposed by hereditary. Amyotrophic lateral sclerosis exhibits mixed presentation of upper motor neuron and lower motor neuron symptoms which is the diagnostic criteria.

Clinical Presentation

- It mostly begins as asymmetrical and unilateral involvement.
- The person experiences difficulty in precision activities of hand.
- There is weakness, wasting, and cramping of the small muscles of the hand .
- As the disease progresses the forearm, upper arm, and shoulder musculatures are also involved.
- In the later stages the disease becomes symmetrical and there is bilateral involvement.
- The lower extremities shown signs of spasticity with brisk reflexes and positive Babinski sign.
- Wasting is primarily of the interossei and lumbricals as compared to long flexors giving rise to a skeletal hand appearance.
- The sphincter functions and abdominal reflexes remain spared in most cases.
- Very rarely the progression may be in a different form where the disease manifests itself in the form of *Crural Amyotrophy* in which there is weakness and wasting of the Pretibial muscles which then progresses to involve the other muscles by involving the trunk and abdominal muscles first before affecting the muscles of the extremities.

Progressive Muscular Atrophy

Clinical Features

- Male population are involved more at a ratio of 4 : 1.
- There is strictly lower motor neuron type of presentation beginning in the hands.
- There is gross weakness, wasting, fasciculations in the hand and then the disease progresses to involve the other parts of the extremities as well as the lower limbs.
- In the lower limbs peritibial muscles are involved and the patient ends up having a "Foot Drop".

- Unlike amyotrophic lateral sclerosis, this disease progresses very gradually up to 10 to 15 years and there are no signs of corticospinal tract involvement.

Progressive Bulbar Palsy

In this condition there is involvement of motor nuclei in the lower brainstem.

Clinical Features

- There is primary involvement of the bulbar muscles and hence the jaw muscles, facial muscles, tongue, larynx and pharynx are affected.
- Due to involvement of the bulbar muscles the patient suffers from dysphagia, dysarthria etc.
- As the muscles of mastication and deglutition are affected the food particles get stuck to one corner of the mouth.
- Fibrillation of tongue is very common.
- Weakness of the pharyngeal muscles causes improper pushing of food particles into esophagus giving rise to chocking.
- In the later stages there may be upper motor neuron type of involvement and jaw jerk may be exaggerated giving rise to strong blinking of eye and wide opening of the mouth that gives rise to "Bull Dog" appearance.
- Death in this condition is mainly due to respiratory failure and the whole disease progresses within a span of 2 years.

Primary Lateral Sclerosis

This type of motor neuron disease may also have hereditary predisposition and there is only upper motor neuron type of presentation.

Clinical Features

- As the diseases have only involvement of both the corticospinal and corticobulbar paths it gives rise to upper motor neuron types of presentation in the extremities and face.
- There is no fasciculation and amyotrophy in this condition.
  Pathologically there is severe loss of pyramidal cells in precentral gyrus with degeneration of corticospinal and corticobulbar fibers.

Pathology of MND

The disease affects primarily the upper motor neuron (pyramidal cells, corticospinal tract and corticobulbar fibers) and the lower motor neuron (cranial nerve nuclei in brainstem and anterior horn cells. The affected neuron shrinks and they are covered with a thick layer of pigmented lipids and this process is called as lipofuscin. Because of the affection of the motor neurons there is severe wasting and weakness of corresponding muscles.

The main feature of this disorder is involvement of selective neuronal cells. The sensory apparatus, the part of the brain involved in controlled and coordinated movement as well as the part of the brain involved in cognition remain absolutely intact.

Diagnosis

The diagnosis of this disorder can be made on three typical features:
1. Involvement restricted to upper motor and lower motor neuron.
2. Whether there is any involvement of other neurons apart from motor neurons (There is no sensory loss in MND).
3. Presence of conduction block in electrophysiological study will rule out the chances of this condition.

The disease has to be differentiated from syringomyelia, intramedullary tumor and cervical myelopathy. These have sensory involvement but have similar picture as in motor neuron disease.

Treatment

The etiology is not known. Motor neuron disease doesn't have a cure. Physical therapy aims to keep the patient as active as possible within the limits of pathology.

• As the disease has a poor prognosis, the patient may be made to understand in the correct fashion regarding his illness and the precaution he needs to take. False hope should never be given to the patient. The therapist is a part of the rehabilitation team as a whole and hence he should be able to find assistance from members of other discipline in the rehabilitation team for various needs of the patient.

• Gentle active exercises should be given in order to maintain the range of motion and as well as to maintain the strength. Irrespective of the type of paresis, whether it is spastic or flaccid or a combination the patient is encouraged to perform regular exercises. Spasticity of some muscles do help the patient to maintain functional independency for a long time. The patient should be encouraged to move his limb actively throughout the day in as full range of motion as possible either independently or with some assistance. This needs to be done regularly.

- Passive range of motion and gentle stretching also helps in maintaining the range as well maintain the circulation in the area. However passive maneuver should be started only when the limb cannot be moved at all and when the muscles fail to contract with the patient's voluntary efforts.
- Self stretching is taught to the patient to get rid of the cramps which he is likely to get.
- No form of vigorous restricted exercises should be given as they give rise to increased fatiguability and cramps which in longer run can cause more damage than benefit to the patient.
- The patient should be kept as mobile as possible through walking or standing for as long as possible. To assist walking assistance by some relatives or attainder is sufficient, sometimes the patient may need a stick or tripod. Some patient walk despite having gross weakness of antigravity muscles by using various compensatory methods which should not be discouraged.
- Secondary complication in the form of pressure sores and contractures should be avoided and when the person goes into respiratory failure, chest physiotherapy becomes necessary. The therapist should make all sincere efforts to maintain the chest expansion of the patient by teaching and supervising breathing exercises. Vigorous chest physiotherapy technique are generally avoided as they are too painful for the patient and he may not tolerate it. Once the patient is on ventilator and needs clearance of airway the chest physiotherapy is administered little more vigorously.
- Light weighted orthosis may be given for certain patient to gain stability at the joints that may help the patient in being functionally independent for a longer time. Lower limb orthosis like above knee orthosis helps the patient to achieve stability at the knee and ankle which enables weight bearing and gait easier for the patient. Similarly giving a knuckle bender or cockup splint for the upper limb depending upon the involvement can enable the patient to be functionally independent.

- Proper positioning of the patient is necessary because once the limbs become weaker and emaciated it becomes increasing difficult to maintain the upright position. This difficulty is noted in standing, sitting in wheelchair or sitting in bed hence proper positioning is necessary. In order to minimize the effect of gravity on the body the patient should be inclined back from the vertical. Assistance of pillows is necessary for providing him with comfortable position.
- Psychological counseling is very essential to prevent the patient from going into a state of depression and to keep his motivation level high.

Some therapist believes in maintaining the muscle property by giving stimulation which is controversial and is not recommended by the author.

TRANSVERSE MYELITIS

Transverse myelitis is an acute or subacute monophasic usually inflammatory disorder of the spinal cord affecting considerable extent transversely but longitudinally limited to 1 or 2 segments of the spinal cord.

Etiology

It is a postinfectious disorder of the spinal cord that is seen following an episode of influenza, mumps, measles or infections caused by Epstein-Barr virus. However the disease is not obvious at the time of infection but occurs as the infection tapers off. It can occur after infection like smallpox, rabies, etc.

Pathogenesis

It is not a result of direct effect of virus on the spinal cord but is an autoimmune response of the body which gets provoked by infection.

Pathology

There is affection of white as well as gray matter. The spinal cord appear edematous, hyperemic and infiltrated by inflammatory cells.

Clinical Features

- The onset is usually acute or subacute
- Disease usually starts either at back or neck area and is usually localized.

- The spine becomes very tender around the affected area
- Sensory loss: The person may have either altered sensation like paresthesia or loss of sensation which begins in the distal part of the leg and ascends upwards similar to the one in GBS. However unlike GBS there is a sensory level, below which there is completed loss of sensation and above the lesion there is normal sensation. Between this normal and abnormal zone there may be a zone of hypersensitivity in some patients.
- Motor loss: The motor symptoms usually is similar to that in acute traumatic paraplegia with a stage of spinal shock during which the tone is lost and there is areflexia but after some days of spinal shock the tone gradually begins to build up and the reflexes reappear. The babinski sign also becomes positive in the patient at this stage. In case Babinski sign fails to become positive then it indicates necrosis involving multiple segments.
- Sphincter disturbances: During the stage of spinal shock there is atonic bladder but after the stage of spinal shock the patient has automatic type of bladder if the lesion is above the spinal reflex center for micturition.

Differential Diagnosis

- Multiple sclerosis
- Devic's syndrome which starts with optic neuritis
- Systemic lupus erythematosus
- Behcet's syndrome.
  The disease should be distinguished from the above conditions which is done as under:

Multiple Sclerosis

The distinguishing character are remission and exacerbations, affections of more than two areas of CNS and also involvement of optic nerve.

Devic's Syndrome

This is also called as Neuromyelitic optica. It starts with bilateral optic neuritis and is more commonly seen in Asians.

SLE or Systemic Lupus Erythematosus

In addition to neurologic involvement person has rashes over cheeks, skin (butterfly type), arthralgia, myalgia, and renal involvement.

Behcet's Syndrome

Predominant pyramidal tract involvement and psychiatric disturbances along with eye and genital lesions.

Treatment

Medical treatment consists of glucocorticoids given with IV methylprednisolone. Physiotherapy treatment is same as that of paraplegias both in flaccid and spastic stage.

SPINAL ARACHNOIDITIS

Arachnoiditis of the spinal cord is a non-specific inflammatory disease of the arachnoid membrane which is characterized pathologically by opacification and thickening of the arachnoid membrane with adhesion or adherence to the dura mater and manifested clinically through roots or radicular signs and symptoms and in severe cases even with cord compression.

Causes

1. *Surgical procedures*
   a. Extradural causes like laminectomy, disectomy, spinal fusion.
   b. Intradural causes like excision of intramedullary tumors, rhizotomy, etc.
2. *Injected agents:* Spinal anesthesia, injection of contrast medium and intradural steroids.
3. Space occupying lesions like neurofibromatosis.
4. Infections like tuberculosis and syphilis.
5. Intrathecal hemorrhage.

Pathology

Inflammatory changes in the arachnoid membrane causes hyperemia opacification thickening and increase in the number of inflammatory cells in the affected area because of inflammation. There is accumulation of exudates which causes adhesions between the fibrous tissues and also between the nerve roots and the thecal sac. There is proliferation of fibrocytes that causes formation of collagen fibers around the nerve roots. Because of this encapsulation of nerve roots from all these areas hypoxia sets in leading to atrophy of the nerve roots.

Clinical Features

- Arachnoiditis is usually seen in 40 to 60 years of age but rarely below 20 years.
- Onset: It can be acute or sometimes it may take months
- Pain: Pain is usually localized type with a burning character. Later the pain starts radiating down the lower limb due to nerve root irritation.
- Paresthesia: This also takes place due to irritation of the sensory nerve roots
- Sensory loss: This occurs when the sensory nerve roots get completely blocked
- Muscle weakness with atrophy: Although the anatomy of the motor nerve roots make them less prone to get compressed, it can happen in the later stage which will then give rise to weakness and wasting of the corresponding muscles.

Signs

The common signs of arachnoiditis are:
- Paraspinal muscle spasm
- Tenderness
- Scoliosis
- Areflexia
- Sphincter disturbances

Investigations

MRI, lumbar puncture, CSF examination shows increase in protein concentration.

Management

The medical management usually consists of corticosteroids in acute stage of inflammation. NSAID for relief of pain and inflammation.

Surgical management consists of Rhizotomy in cases of unbearable pain.

Surgical decompression for removal of cyst.

Physiotherapy management comprises of
1. Moist heat mainly for reducing the muscle spasm.
2. SSF also relieves pain by reducing spasm and by increasing the blood supply to the area.

3. In case of radiating pain due to involvement of nerve roots the patient may be treated with TENS. Even in cases of paresthesia TENS is usually used.

4. Laser has been found to reduce the inflammation and also break the adhesion in the deep seated structures which helps in setting free the irritation on the nerve roots thereby relieving the discomforts of the patient.

5. Active exercises like static exercises for the abdominus, back extensor, gluteus and quadriceps helps in reducing pain in the initial stages and also maintains the tone in the muscles.

6. Dynamic exercises may be started once the pain level comes within the patient's tolerance level. These exercises may be continued by the patient throughout the life for preventing any chances of recurrence.

7. SLR: Active and passive SLR is given to lengthen the neural structures and relieve the tension in them. This is a type of neural mobilization that helps in relieving the signs of radiculopathy.

8. Gait training in cases of muscular weakness.

CERVICAL MYELOPATHY

It is a chronic pathological disorder of the spinal cord caused due to compression of the spinal cord by various degenerative changes. The cause of compression can be osteophytes, thickened and calcified ligaments, disc prolapse and transverse bar.

Signs and Symptoms

- *Age:* Condition is usually seen in a person who is more than 40 years.
- *Onset:* The condition usually occurs gradually or insidiously, infact it begins as a mild negligible pain which is often ignored by many patient and then progresses very slowly before causing major signs. The condition usually runs a very chronic course.
- *Neck stiffness:* Restriction is more of lateral flexion and lateral rotation and later even of flexion and extension.
- *Neck pain:* Pain felt on posterior aspect of neck spreading to supraspinous area and increases with any neck movements.
- *Brachialgia:* The patient experiences pain along the upper extremities which could be stabbing or dull ache in character

and could radiate to the shoulder, elbow or even to the tip of the finger. Rarely the patient may perceive the sensory symptoms as burning in character.

- *Sensory loss:* It depends upon site of compression. If there is posterolateral compression then the pain and temperature sensations are the first to get involved. In case the compression is purely posterior then the patient will have affection of the joint position sensation, vibration sensation and there will be positive Romberg's sign. This type of sensory loss mimics the type seen in tabes dorsalis.
- *Motor symptoms:* Usually motor signs may be first seen in the lower extremity due to the anatomical position of the corticospinal tracts. Lower extremity shows signs of spasticity. Patient complains of heaviness or stiffness in the lower limbs and the deep tendon reflexes are exaggerated or brisk. Babinski may be positive. In the later stages patient may complain of difficulty in micturition and over a prolonged time without proper treatment the patient may even become bedridden due to quadriparesis.
- *Vertibular basilar artery syndrome:* Compression of this artery can cause giddiness or sudden blackouts during certain neck movements as a result of compression of the vertibular artery at the cervical level.

Pathology

With age there is calcification of ligaments and intervertebral disc are covered with fibrous tissues. Whenever roots are compressed the dural sleeves is thickened and the underlying root fibers are damaged. The main pathological changes are seen at the site of cord compression which is represented by focal demyelination, necrosis and loss of nerve cells.

Pathogenesis

The lower cervical spine is more affected due to increased mobility that puts more stress upon the lower cervical spine. The process that causes cord damage is compression of the cord followed by ischemia. However these are not the only factors that accounts for severe symptoms shown by patients. The osteophytes encroaching the spinal canal causes damage to spinal cord every time the cervical spine is moved which in turn increases the friction between the spinal cord and the osteophytes. Moreover whenever there is extension movement of the neck the ligamentous flavum infolds within the spinal canal causing damage to the cord and pain to the patient. Since in a degenerative case there is already compression on the anterior part. This infolding of ligamentum flavum adds on to the compression thereby making the entire situation more complex. The presence of vascular insufficiency due to compression of vertebral artery can further worsen the situation.

Diagnosis

Presence of clear cut clinical features of cervical spondylosis confirmed through X-rays, MRI and myelogram should make the diagnosis simple. The other diseases that can give rise to similar picture are myopathies, neuropathies and amyotrophic lateral sclerosis.

Treatment

In the initial stages conservative treatment with analgesics and physiotherapy treatment is effective and can prevent further complication. Cervical collars are prescribed to prevent secondary damage to cord during movement. Pain relief may be obtained by use to modalities like IFT, TENS, moist heat, etc. However they may fail to show long term benefits and hence when the patient starts showing compromise in the neurological structures surgery is undertaken. The usual surgery done is laminectomy for decompressing the nerve.

TUMORS OF THE SPINAL CORD

Tumors or neoplasm or space occupying lesions are classified broadly into *intramedullary* and *extramedullary* tumors.

Intramedullary tumors are those present within the substance of the spinal cord. It could be either a primary tumors or a metastasis. Extramedullary tumors are those present outside the substance of the spinal cord. They can be further divided into intradural and extradural.

The intradural ones are meningioma, ones that arise from the nerve roots and the extradural ones arises from epidural substances and vertebral bodies.

Classification of Tumors

Extradural	Intradural	Intramedullary
In Infants		
Neuroblastoma	Meningioma	Ependymoma
Ganglioneuroma	Neurofibroma	
Sarcoma	Angioma	
In Adults		
Ganglioneuroma	Meningioma	Glioma
Sarcoma	Neurofibroma	Ependymoma
Chondroma		

Symptoms

Tumors of the spinal cord can give rise to any one of the following symptoms:
- Sensorimotor spinal tract syndrome
- Radicular spinal cord syndrome
- Intramedullary syringomyelia syndrome

Sensori motor spinal tract syndrome: This symptom begins in a very gradual manner. It usually starts with pain and tenderness at the affected spinous process. The spinal tract are the first to get affected and as a result the person shows altered sensation or dysesthesia. If the spinothalamic tract is fully compressed there will be total loss of pain and temperature sensation in the affected part of the body.

Motor signs and symptoms are usually of upper motor neuron type due to compression of the corticospinal tract and it depends upon the level and extent of involvement. The compression caused by extradural tumors when relieved leads to almost complete recovery which is always in a reverse order (which Means the part affected first will be the last to recover).

Radicular spinal cord syndrome: This symptom also begins in the form of pain and is usually of radiating character from the spine and is intensified by activities like coughing, sneezing, straining and from prolonged recumbency. There will also be tingling numbness and paresthesia along affected nerve roots, areflexia and lower motor type of muscular paralysis due to involvement of motor nerve roots. Along with the radicular signs and symptoms, the person will also have symptoms due to compression of the spinal cord and these are spastic paraparesis, loss of pain and temperature sensation, loss of sensation by the posterior column and even bowel–bladder disturbances.

Intramedullary synringomyelia syndrome: The signs and symptoms are similar to syringomyelia which is already explained in the beginning of this chapter.

Thus there is initially involvement of pain and temperature fibers followed by involvement of the anterior horn cells at the level and later on by involvement of the corticospinal fibers and other sensory tracts.

The pain which arises from spinal cord tumor has to be distinguished from pain having an organic origin. Pain due to tumor in the spinel is usually associated with tenderness of the spine and is related to activities like coughing, sneezing along with associated findings like tingling numbness, paresthesia or loss of sensation along the particular dermatome. Also there will be motor signs and symptoms along with altered deep tendon reflexes. However one should not come to a conclusion only based on clinical grounds.

Investigations

The diagnosis of spinal cord syndrome can be confirmed with investigations like CT scan, MRI, myelogram and CSF examination to be carried out in order to come to a proper diagnosis.

Management

Surgical intervention is a must in most of the cases of spinal cord tumors. Extramedullary tumors can be excised and recovery is always good, whereas intramedullary tumors requires decompression like laminectomy followed by radiation. The prognosis is always better if operative procedure is carried out in initial stages before neurological deficit becomes very obvious. Postoperative physiotherapy is very essential to obtain maximum functional output following the surgery.

MULTIPLE SCLEROSIS

Although multiple sclerosis doesn't necessarily be limited as spinal cord disease it is put in this chapter because one of the areas that it has a predilection is the dorsal column of the spinal cord.

Multiple sclerosis is a demyelinating disease affecting the white matter of the central nervous system. Although the lesion generally appears to be disseminated (hence it is also called as disseminated sclerosis) there are certain areas which are more prone like the cerebrum, cerebellar peduncles, brainstem and dorsal spinal cord. The lesion tends to be more or less symmetrical. The common characteristic clinical and pathological findings that are observed in multiple sclerosis are paralysis, intentional tremor, scanning speech and nystagmus. These findings were first observed by Dr Jean Charcot and hence it is termed as *Charcot's triad.*

Multiple sclerosis is a very unpredictable disease with a characteristic *exacerbation and remission.*

Clinical Features

- Age: The common age group involved is 15 to 40 years.
- Progression: The condition can take different mode of progression. It can be Benign where it starts suddenly, progresses slowly and has complete remission or it can be Exacerbation–Remission with gradual progression and partial remission or it could be Remission—Progressive with incomplete remission along with disability or it can be Progressive with no remission.
- Sensory deficit: Patient can have sensory complains like tingling numbness, loss of sensation carried by dorsal column, hyperpathia (hypersensitiveness), dysesthesia (altered sensation) and even trigeminal neuralgia.
- Motor symptoms: The patient may have spasticity due to involvement of the pyramidal fibers along with generalized weakness or paresis.
- Reflexes: The plantar response show Babinski positive, with hyper-excitable deep tendon jerks and sometimes clonus. The other superficial reflexes are absent.

- The patient can show signs of cerebellar involvement like intentional tremor, dysmetria, dysdiadochokinesia, incoordination, and nystagmus.
- The patient also feel a sense of fatigability and show reduced fitness level.
- Visual disturbances like optic neuritis, central scotoma or blind spot may be noted.
- Bowel and bladder dysfunction like urgency, precipitancy, or retention of urine may be seen.
- Cognitive disturbances like reduced attention span, decreased ability to learn, euphoria, fluctuation in mood or emotion, etc. are observed.

The patient may have secondary manifestations like anxiety or depression, musculoskeletal problems like stiffness, osteoporosis, etc. cardiorespiratory deconditioning, renal complications and GIT complications.

Management

- Sensory retraining: Various sensory stimulation like tapping, vibration, stroking, and hacking can be used to bring about sensory reeducation. Object of various size, shape, textures and weight may be used to stimulate sensation in these patients. The patient may be advised to use visual sensation as a compensatory mechanism or loss of tactile and proprioceptive sensations. TENS may be used for the tingling sensation. Various techniques of home adaptation is necessary to increase the visual input to help the patient in overcoming the blurred vision. Regular inspection of the body parts is necessary to check for any sores or wound. The patient should also be instructed to maintain good skin hygiene so as to prevent any chances of infection.
- The patient can be given relief from pain by using electrical modalities like TENS, IFT or even hot packs to relieve muscle spasm.
- Spasticity can be reduced by prolonged icing, sustained stretching, gentle passive movement, weight bearing exercises, biofeedback, etc.
- Mobility and flexibility exercise for the joint is essential to prevent stiffness. Stretching of biarticular muscles of the lower and upper limb is necessary. Gentle passive movement also helps to main-

tain range of motion at all joints. PNF techniques like hold relax, contract relax helps in lengthening tight muscles.

- Management of paresis and fatigability can be achieved by improving the strength and endurance of the muscles. Resisted exercises based upon the capacity of the patient may be given. Weight bearing activities helps in increasing the strength and endurance of various postural muscles. In order to overcome fatigue the patient may be taught some energy conservation techniques.
- Coordination exercises needs to be given to overcome incoordination.
- Gait training initially with support and later on without support should be carried out. Infact some patients may need some orthosis to improve their walking abilities.
- Good deep breathing exercises and aerobic exercises needs to be given to correct cardiorespiratory deconditioning.

SELF-ASSESSING QUESTIONS

Long and Short Essay

- Explain the PT management of patient with syringomyelia extending from C5 to C7 area of the spinal cord.
- Describe the clinical features and management of syringomyelia.
- Describe the management of multiple sclerosis patient.
- Describe the clinical features and management of multiple sclerosis.
- Discuss the clinical features of various types of motor neuron diseases.
- Discuss the clinical features and management of cervical myelopathy.
- Discuss about arachnoiditis.
- Describe the PT management of acute transverse myelitis at T8 spinal segment in acute and chronic stage.
- Describe the clinical features and management of case of transverse myelitis at T12 spinal segment in spastic stage.

Short Answers

- What is brown Sequard syndrome?
- What is posterior cord syndrome?
- What is central cord syndrome?

- What is anterior cord syndrome?
- What is anal sparing?
- What is brachial amyotrophy?
- What is stretch reflex?
- Define tone.

10

ETIOLOGY

Mechanism of the injury that can cause damage to the vertebrae with a resultant damage to the cord is usually a hyperflexion with rotation movement. Extension with rotation is less likely to cause damage to the cord.

Injuries to the spinal cord can be caused to:

1. *Fractures or fracture with dislocation:* Hyperflexion with rotation or direct force giving rise to horizontal displacement of vertebra. Fracture dislocation of the cervical vertebrae is usually due to violent sudden hyperflexion forces however rarely a sudden extension movement can cause the damage. Thoracic spine damage can occur due to direct blow as seen in violent flexion injuries when a person is in sitting position. Thoracolumbar and lumbar spine fracture or fracture dislocation is caused due to fall from a height and is usually associated with a calcaneus fracture.
2. *Sports injuries:* For example, diving can cause injury to the cervical spine. Even whiplash injuries are common due to various motor sports like Formula race, etc.
3. *Industrial injuries:* Fall of a heavy object on the head, neck or back especially in people whose job demands lifting heavy weight like porters, laborers in tyre company, etc. are very prone for this type of damage.
4. *Stab injury:* Very common in India due to riots or gang wars.
5. *Gunshot injuries:* The percentage of this type of injuries has increased over recent years.
6. *Surgical procedures:* Surgeries done in and around the spinal cord can cause damage to it.

Fracture or fracture dislocation can be caused either due to collision of a heavy object over the head or directly over the spine. It can also be caused due to collision of the head against a hard but static object. Manipulation in a incorrect manner commonly caused by non-professional like Saloons can cause damage to the spine. In rural India especially in the costal area spinal cord injury is common due to fall from a coconut tree which causes severe damage to the spinal cord.

PATHOLOGY

Soon after spinal cord injury, some vascular and biochemical changes occurs which leads to infarction which in turn leads to necrosis. Infarction could be due to either direct injury to the spinal cord arteries or due to certain biochemical events that leads to hypoxia which causes edema and that finally leads to infarction. Any trauma to the spinal cord leads to release in non-epinephrine which is a vasoconstrictor causing infarction.

CLINICAL FEATURES

Immediately following an acute injury to the spinal cord there is a stage of Spinal Shock:

Spinal shock is a state of areflexia characterized by loss of tone, loss of reflexes and total inactivity. The cause of this stage is not fully understood. It is believed that an abrupt cessation of physiological excitatory state due to sudden loss of connections between the higher centers and the spinal cord could be the cause of spinal shock. The period of the spinal shock can last for 24 hours to weeks but is usually resolved within 24 to 48 hours. The first indicator of the resolving of spinal shock is the presence of bulbo-cavernous reflex. It can be elicited both in males and females. In males the organ stimulated is penis and in females it is the clitoris. This reflex can be positive even weeks before the deep tendon reflexes are elicited. However presence of bulbocavernous reflex without any emergence or presence of tone or any reflex months after injury indicates severe damage to spinal cord and is usually a bad prognostic sign.

After the stage of spinal shock has passed the various neurological deficits starts manifesting which commonly consists of the following:
• *Motor deficit and sensory loss:* This depends upon certain features of the lesion like neurological level of lesion, completeness or extent of lesion, symmetry of lesion and sacral sparing or root escape.

- *Loss of thermoregulatory functions:* Due to damage to spinal cord, the ascending tract that carries information regarding the peripheral temperature to the hypothalamus is cut hence the hypothalamus does not receive proper information regarding environmental temperature due to which it is unable to control cutaneous blood flow and sweating. As a result there is no vasodilatation or constriction with response to head or cold environment. Sometimes in cases of incomplete lesion you may get spotty sweating in a localized area below level of lesion. The disability is more pronounced in places where there is frequent fluctuation in atmospheric temperature.

- *Respiratory dysfunction:* Any injury to the spinal cord that affects second, third and fourth cervical spinal area causes involvement of the phrenic nerve as a result of which there is denervation of the diaphragm muscles which is the main inspiratory muscle. These patients may need ventilatory support or phrenic nerve stimulator. Involvement of the thoracic spine causes involvement of the corresponding intercoastals muscles which definitely will cause difficulty in breathing but the patient does not have to totally depend on artificial ventilation. The severity of dysfunction will depend upon the level of lesion, preserved respiratory muscles, associated injuries to the chest wall and the patient's previous respiratory status.

  On the contrary, if the lesion is in the lumbar spine then there is paraplegia without respiratory dysfunction.

  The affection of the respiratory system represents a fatal feature of the spinal cord injury. Death of the person is usually caused due to pulmonary embolism or even bronchiectasis. Inability to cough or perform forceful expulsion of air causes severe retention of fluid or secretions and hence there is consequent pulmonary infection.

- *Spasticity:* Spasticity is a state of hyperactivity where you have hypertonicity, hyperreflexia and clonus. Spasticity usually increases during first six months after spinal injury and reaches a plateau by the end of first year. It can be precipitated or aggravated by positional changes, cutaneous stimulation, fecal impaction, renal and bladder stones, blockage of catheter, urinary retention, tight clothing or decubitus ulcer. Mild to moderate spasticity allows movement to take place and infact the patient can learn to precipitate spasticity of certain muscles in order to gain functional independence. Severe spasticity on the other hand comes in the way of rehabilitation and prevents functional independence.

• *Bladder dysfunction:* This is one of the most common clinical features of the spinal cord injuries. The chances of complication in the form of urinary tract infections and calculi are very high if proper medical attention is not provided in initial stages.

Soon after any spinal cord injury during stage of spinal shock there is presence of atonic bladder or flaccid bladder in which due to loss of tone the bladder acts as a balloon and goes on accommodating as much urine as possible till the point of overflow incontinence. The main aim of medical management is to prevent any secondary complications in the form of urinary tract infections or stones. Thus continuous catherization is given.

Automatic or Reflex bladder is seen when there is damage to the spinal cord above the micturition center which is S2,S3,S4. Since the reflex center is intact reflex emptying of bladder takes place soon after the pressure inside the bladder reaches a particular level beyond which it exerts stretch upon the detrusor muscles. This reflex emptying can be stimulated by use of various sensory input like kneading, tapping, stroking suprapubic area or by pinching, pulling of hair over the lower abdominal, pubic or inner thigh area.

Autonomous bladder or areflex bladder: Whenever there is damage to the S2, S3,S4 segments of the spinal cord it causes interruption of the reflex pathway thereby leading to flaccid autonomous areflex bladder that causes overflow incontinence. Voiding can still be accomplished by bringing about strong contraction of the abdominal muscles by process known as Valsalva or Credé's maneuver.

Bladder Training Program can be Achieved by Two Methods

Intermittent catheterization: The main aim of bladder training is to establish a proper process of voiding and make the patient catheter free as early as possible. It is very essential that the person learn voiding at a regular and predictable interval. Firstly the fluid intake of the patient should be restricted to 1800 to 2000 ml per day. The person should be advised to stop fluid intake towards the late evening hours so as to prevent need for catheterization at night or nocturia. The person's fluid intake has to be monitored at 180-200 ml per hour. Initially the person is catheterized after every four hours. Before catheterization the person is asked to stimulate voiding voluntarily following which catheter is introduced to drain out the residual urine which is measured. As the bladder is training program becomes more and more effective the person learns to void voluntarily and the amount of residual urine gets reduced and frequency of catheterization also reduces.

Timed voiding program: The person's pattern of incontinence has to be studied along with pattern of fluid intake. This enables patient to established a new pattern of fluid intake and voiding program so that the person can make use of the techniques and void at a regular interval to get rid of overflow and catheterization. However it is necessary to know that not all bladder training programs are successful and many times the person has to be catheterized permanently.

Condom catheters are advised in males to prevent urinary tract infection whereas in males indwelling catheter is the only option.

(The other types of neurogenic bladder are cortical bladder which comprises of hesitancy and precipitancy, motor bladder and sensory bladder. Cortical bladder occurs due to lesion to the paracentral lobule of the cerebral cortex. The cortical control over the pons is lost hence the patient is not able to initiate micturition when the conditions are favorable but micturates when the conditions are not favorable. This condition can be treated by either catheterization or by avoiding fluid intake when the patient has to go to some social gathering.

Sensory bladder is the one in which the sensory fibers of the reflex arc are damaged like in conditions like tabes dorsalis or diabetic neuropathy hence patient doesn't have the sensation of bladder filling. This patient can be taught to recognize bladder filling by appreciating alternative sensation like discomfort in the abdomen, excessive sweating, etc. Forceful voiding can then be achieved by Valsalva maneuver or Credé's maneuver.

Motor bladder is the one in which the sensory fibers of the reflex pathway is intact but the motor fibers are damaged like in cases of polio hence the patient is not able to voluntarily micturate although he has the sensation of bladder filling. Management is same as above using Valsalva and Credé's maneuver).

Sexual Dysfunction

The sympathetic supply for sexual function which brings about ejaculation is T12 to L1 whereas the parasympathetic supply which brings about erection is from S2, S3, S4 segments. In spinal cord injuries above S2, S3,S4, the physiological erection remains intact in 90 percent of patients. Psychological erection may be possible in incomplete lesion of spinal cord. In lower motor neuron lesion due to damage to reflex arc the physiological erections are lost but psychological erection may remain intact if the lesion is incomplete. Ejaculation is possible if the lesion is below the L2 area of the spinal cord irrespective of whether the erection is present or not. However in cases of complete lesion above L2 area ejaculation may be affected.

COMPLICATION OF SPINAL CORD INJURIES

Pressure Sores

Certain area in the body is subjected to continuous pressure as the amount of protective tissues between the skin and the bones are less or absent. These areas are heels, malleolus, and head of fibula, sacrum, spine of scapula, greater trochanter, ischial tuberosity, elbow and even the occiput. Continuous pressure impairs the blood supply to the area hence it becomes dry and break up causing ulceration, the continues lack of blood only makes the wound worse and worser without letting it get healed. Under normal circumstances the hydrostatic pressure within the capillaries keep them patent but in an immobilized patient constant pressure overcomes the constant hydrostatic pressure of the capillaries leading to their closure which causes the interruption in the blood supply to this sensitive area. Thus the person who is continuously immobilized has a tendency to develop pressure sores at those areas, which are continuously subjected to pressure.

Tightness, Contractures and Deformity

Soft tissues across a joint when maintained in a shortened position for a long time may lead to contractures. Muscles are first to be affected followed by ligaments and capsules. Certain muscles in the body are more prone to develop these complications namely the shoulder adductors, elbow flexors, pronators, long flexors of the hand, hip and knee flexors, pronators, long flexors of hand, hip and knee flexors and plantar flexors. These contractures are developed due to muscular imbalance, faulty position maintained for a long time and the influence of gravitational force.

Deep vein thrombosis: In a patient with spinal cord injury due to lack of mobility there is stagnation of blood. Research studies has shown that when the blood remains stagnated for more than 10 to 12 hours it leads to clotting of blood within the vessels. The deep vein thrombosis could prove to be a very fatal complication because of its tendency to cause Pulmonary and Cerebral embolism. To prevent this one has to inspect the body parts at least once in a day. Earlier ready-made stockings were available to exert pressure peripherally so that the blood is pushed from the peripheral to the proximal area. However due to rapid wasting that follows a spinal cord injury causes the pressure exerted by the stockings to gradually become reduced hence these days elastocrepe bandages are used. Also intravenous heparin is of great use in preventing and overcoming DVT as long as the person is immobile.

Osteoporosis

In a spinal cord injury patient the calcium metabolism below the site of injury is affected. Normally there is a good balance between bone formation by osteoblasts and resorption of bones by osteoclastic activity. However inpatient with spinal cord injury, the bone formation remains intact but the absorption of calcium into the bones is reduced. Thus the patient develops osteoporosis. This is primarily due to lack of weight bearing by the person. Moreover as the calcium formed is not absorbed from the blood into the bones there is increase in the concentration of calcium in the blood which is called as hypocalcemia which also leads to increase in the calcium concentration in the urine and is termed as hypercalciuria. The increase in the calcium concentration in the urine can in turn give rise to abdominal pain, urinary retention and even urinary stone formation.

Autonomous Dysreflexia

It is an acute sympathetic discharge observed in a spinal cord injury patient with lesion over T5 spinal segments and is characterized by hypertension, profuse sweating, headache, flushing of face, nasal congestion, piloerection and bradycardia. This reflex usually occurs in response to any noxious stimuli. The stimuli can be catheterization, urinary stones, tight clothing, pressure sores, bowel or bladder distension. It can also occur due to any form of tactile stimulation.

Urinary Tract Infection and Urinary Calculi

Due to urinary retention in the spinal cord injury patient there is growth of bacteria primarily due to the presence of an indwelling catheter which acts as a main source of entrance for the bacteria. Thus the patient invariably suffers from urinary tract infections if proper precautions are not taken in the initial stages itself. Moreover the presence of urinary retention causes influx of urine back into the kidney causing infection of the kidney. Also due to stagnation of urine combine with hypercalciuria the patient becomes more prone to develop urinary stone or calculi. Although the incidence of calcium stone is more, one should know that other salts like phosphates, carbonates, magnesium can also cause formation of stones in spinal cord injury patients.

Heterotrophic Bone Formation

This means formation of bones within the muscles however unlike myositis ossifica ons where there is bone formation within the muscle belly in this case the bone formation takes place either in the tendon or in the connective tissues of the muscles. This type of changes are seen in spinal cord injury patients after 4 to 6 months following the onset although radiological findings will remain negative. It can be treated either with drug therapy like diphosphates, gentle passive movements or surgical intervention.

Pain Syndromes

This is quite a common complication following spinal cord injury. The source of pain can be traumatic (due to the initial trauma), radicular (arising from the nerve roots), spinal cord pain (due to dyesthesia which is altered sensation), and musculoskeletal (due to severe stress put on the joints of the upper limb commonly the shoulder joint).

Gastrointestinal Complication

Prolonged immobility or reduced immobility interferes with peristaltic activity and bowel movements causing the development of constipation and peptic ulcer.

MANAGEMENT

Management of spinal cord injury is same as that of paraplegia for lumbar and thoracic lesion. Spinal cord injury at the cervical spine needs to be managed as quadriparesis. For quadriparesis upper limb strengthening, intensive chest care and proper wheelchair management is necessary in addition to the management of paraplegia.

SELF-ASSESSING QUESTIONS

- Give clinical features of spinal cord injury.
- Give clinical features and management of spinal cord injury at T10 spinal level.
- Explain the complication following spinal cord injury.
- Explain neurogenic bladder following spinal cord injury.
- Describe different types of neurogenic bladder and give their management.

11

Paraplegia

Paralysis of both the lower limbs without any involvement of the upper limbs is called as Paraplegia.

CAUSES

Upper Motor Neuron Lesion

Intracranial Causes (This Occurs Very Rarely)

- Tumors of the falx cerebri
- Thrombosis of superior sagittal sinus
- Thrombosis of unpaired anterior cerebral artery affecting both leg area.

Spinal Causes

- Subacute combined degeneration of the cord
- Multiple sclerosis
- Acute transverse myelitis
- Motor neuron disease—amyotrophic lateral sclerosis
- Fracture dislocation of the thoracic or lumbar vertebrae
- Epidural abscess
- Vascular causes like hemorrhage, thrombosis, arteriovenous malformation
- Compression of the cord by space occupying lesion
- Radiation myelopathy
- Pott's paraplegia following tuberculosis of the spine
- Hereditary spastic paraparesis.
- Trauma.

Lower Motor Neuron Lesion

- Anterior horn cells lesion in conditions like poliomyelitis, spinal muscular atrophy and motor neuron diseases
- Roots lesion like in cauda equina syndrome

- Peripheral nerve lesion such as in neuropathies, polyneuritis
- Myasthenia gravis
- Muscular conditions like muscular dystrophies, polymyositis
- Spina bifida with myelomeningocele.

CLINICAL PRESENTATION

In lesions that are acute like acute transverse myelitis, there will be a stage of spinal shock. During the stage of shock the tone of the muscles are reduced (flaccid or hypotonicity), the reflexes are absent (areflexia), atonic or flaccid bladder will be seen and hence the patient will be totally dependent on others for his activities of daily living. After the stage of shocked has passed, the lower limbs will present with either upper motor neuron or lower motor neuron type of paralysis depending on the level of lesion. Lesion in the cauda equina will present as typical lower motor neuron type of paralysis. Thoracic or higher lumbar lesion will show lower motor neuron type of picture at the level of lesion and upper motor type of paralysis below the level of lesion. To understand the above statement let us consider that the patient has involvement of L2 and L3 spinal segments. In this case muscles having their root values as L2, L3 like the quadriceps will show lower motor neuron type of lesion whereas muscles with root values that is lower than the above like L5, S1, S2, etc. will show upper motor neuron type of presentation.

Paraplegia in Flexion and Paraplegia in Extension

It depends on intact connections between the reticular formation nuclei and the spinal cord. If the spinal lesion in partial so as to spare the reticulospinal tract, extensor hypertonia predominates. Occasionally flexor withdrawal reflex is elicited on giving noxious stimulus.

If the spinal lesion destroys not only CST but also RST, Flexor withdrawal reflex is freed from its antagonists and shows domination. The involvement of vestibulospinal and rubrospinal tract also determines the presence of paraplegia in flexion or extension.

Complications of Paraplegia

- *Pressure sores:* In case of chronic illness with paraplegia the patient is bed-ridden for a long time. If proper care is not taken patient develops pressure sores which becomes a major complication if infected.

- *Tightness and contractures:* Because of inability of the patient to move the lower limbs, patients lower limbs are positioned under the effect of gravity or under the influence of spasticity. This position if continued for a long time leads to loss of physiological excursion of soft tissues. The patient suffers from tightness, contractures and loss of ROM. If these are not treated in time it will lead to fixed malalignment of joints which eventually will lead to deformity.

- *Impairment of tone:* Depending on the level of lesion the patient presents with either flaccidity seen in lower motor neuron type of lesion or spasticity seen in upper motor neuron type of lesion. Abnormal alteration of tone affects the normal movement of the lower limbs and leads to abnormal gait patterns or loss of ambulation.

- *Osteoporosis:* Without adequate weight bearing imposed on the lower limb bones more and more calcium is released from bones which causes osteoporotic and fragile bones that is prone to have fractures even with trivial trauma.

- *Urinary complication:* The common urinary complications that the patient can develop are urinary tract infection and renal or bladder calculi. Urinary retention or dribbling coupled with poor hygiene increases the chances of infection in the urinary tract. As the patient is bedridden, the absorption of calcium by the bone is reduced. This causes accumulation of calcium in the blood that eventually gets deposited in the kidney causing *Renal calculi.*

- *Respiratory complications:* Higher thoracic level lesion that causes paralysis of respiratory muscles like the intercostals and the abdominal will cause a gross reduction in the vital capacity of the patient. Further more, the weakness of the abdominal muscles causes a very ineffective cough which allows the secretions to get accumulated hence causing secondary infection.

- *Depression:* As the patient is no longer a contributing member in the family, he develops a complexity about himself and hence goes into a state of depression which adds on to his physical disability.

Physiotherapy Management

The aims of the physiotherapy management consists of

a. Prevention of all secondary complications as a result of being bedridden.

b. Restoration of functional independency to the maximum possible limit.
c. Psychological counseling.
d. Social and vocational rehabilitation.
e. Family education and home adaptation.

Counseling

A patient who is depressed cannot cooperate with the therapist which will have a negative effect on the overall rehabilitation of the patient. Hence to gain maximum cooperation from the patient the therapist should give appropriate psychological counseling that will enable the patient to come out of state of depression. The patient needs to be told regarding his condition but at the same time the therapist should try and highlight the positive features contained in the patient even at this stage which in turn will inspire the patient to look at his future in a more convincing manner. However one should not give false hopes to the patient as the expectation of patient may be too high. Interviews or articles of paraplegic patient leading a relatively independent and even successful life will help in changing the patient's mental state.

Maintaining Passive and Active Range of Motion

The patient's lower limb should be moved passively by the therapist through full range of motion if the patient is not able to perform the movement actively. Wherever the patient is likely to put his active efforts to perform the movement, the therapist should encourage it as this will not only maintain the active range but will also help the patient to maintain the properties in his muscles. Passive movements need to be given every two hourly hence the patient's relative attending him should be taught the correct way of handling and giving passive movement without producing undesired movement of the spine. Passive movements helps to maintain the normal physiological length of soft tissues and prevents tightness. It maintains the memory of the movement pattern in the brain which may help in the later stages of recovery. Passive movements also help in reducing spasticity if given in a gentle, slow and rhythmic manner.

Along with passive movements, all the biarticular muscles of the lower limb should be stretched.

Maintenance of Good Bronchial Hygiene

As the patient is totally bedridden it leads to deconditioning of the respiratory system. Moreover in higher cord lesion due to respiratory muscles weakness, the patient needs ventilatory support which further increases the chances of lung infection. Hence proper lung hygiene should be maintained by given proper positioning, nebulization and regular suctioning. If the patient is not on ventilatory support then he should be taught breathing exercises and encouraged doing it every hour.

Care of Skin

Due of constant immobilization the patient can develop pressure sores at certain parts of the body. Certain areas are more susceptible to develop pressure sores like sacrum, heel, lateral aspect of the knee, occiput, etc. Hence prevention and treatment of pressure sores are very important.

Prevention of pressure sores is achieved by undertaking the following measures:

- The patient's attendant as well as the nursing staff should be advised to keep changing the position of the patient every 2 hourly to avoid increase weight bearing pressure on certain body parts especially where the subcutaneous fat is very less.
- Good skin hygiene is maintained by given regular sponge bath and applying talcum powder. As patient with urinary or fecal incontinence are prone to soil the skin around the genital area it is very susceptible to cause skin infection and even urinary tract infection hence more emphasize should be given to these areas to maintain hygiene.
- Bed linen is kept dry and free of creases.
- Beds that bring about a more uniform distribution of body weight should be given. Thus waterbed or airbed is used to equalize the pressure on patient's body and to prevent areas of increase pressure.
- Gently massaging the pressure susceptible areas also increases the circulation in that areas preventing the chances of skin infection.

In case, in spite of the entire preventive measures if the pressure sores do develop then it should be treated at the early stage and the wound should be prevented from getting infected so that the rate of healing is faster. This can be achieved by the following:

- Regular dressing of wound
- Cryotherapy around the wound area to increase circulation
- Infrared therapy over the wound also increases the blood supply to the part and thus helps in faster recovery
- If the wound is infected then UVR can be given
- Laser therapy at appropriate dose can be very effective in healing the sores
- Direct current given at the edges of the sores helps in healing.

Care of Bladder

The patient is taught self-cleaning techniques and intermittent catheterization. For lower motor neuron type of bladder Valsalva maneuver or Credé's maneuver is taught. For patient with upper motor neuron type of bladder Intermittent catheterization technique or timed voiding program may be given.

Active Exercises

As soon as the patient shows signs of active contraction of muscles and active participation, all the exercises that needs active cooperation of the patient should be started. These exercises are essential to make the patient functionally independent. The common exercises which is incorporated into the treatment program consists of Mat exercises, strengthening techniques, weight bearing exercises, normalizing tone in the lower limb, gait training and Transfer activities.

Management of spasticity : Refer Chapter 2.

Mat exercises: To prepare the patient for gait training and erect posture mat exercises play a very important role. These exercises consist of those activities that may help the patient to achieve some functional independency. The activities consist of turning to each sides, rolling and bridging. Similarly in prone position the patient may be given activities such as coming on to forearms, coming on to extended forearms, quadripedal position with the help of some external support, kneeling with support, half kneeling, etc.

Strengthening exercises: These consist of exercises to strengthen the lower limb muscles in case of lower motor neuron type of palsy. Strengthening of the upper limb is essential as this will help the patient to enable efficiency in activities like transferring, use of walking aids like crutch, and also helps in over all functional rehabilitation. Strengthening of trunk muscles is essential for better trunk control and stability which will help in better balancing in sitting or standing. Quadratus lumborum is the most important trunk muscle in case of paraplegia who have got no hip flexors because it enables the patient to hike the pelvis and clear the paretic limb off the ground thus enabling the patient to be ambulant.

- *Use of tilt table:* In the initial stages when there is no trunk stability patient can be trained for weight bearing on lower limbs by using tilt table. In this the patient's trunk and the lower limbs are strapped to the tilt table and then the table is tilted such that the patient is in erect position. Moreover tilt table can also used in the initial stages to prevent the chances of orthostatic hypotension. For preventing hypotension in the initial stages the patient is made to lie on the tilt table and the table is gradually tilted everyday at increasing range so that the autonomous nervous system is made to get conditioned as a result the reflex vasoconstriction can be stimulated in erect position. This will help in preventing or treating orthostatic hypotension.

- *Transfer activities:* To make the patient independent in ADL, it is necessary to train him to use the wheelchair and transfer from and to wheelchair. Easy ways of transfer from bed to wheelchair from wheelchair to low stool and from low stool to floor and back to wheel chair should be taught to patient. The patient also should be trained for balance in sitting position if his trunk muscles are also affected. Patient should also be taught various ways of locomotion in emergency situation like shuffling in sitting position, semicrawling in prone position with the help of weight bearing on the forearm.

- *Gait training:* Paraplegic patient can be made to ambulate with the help of crutches and calipers. There are various types of paraplegic gait that can be taught with the assistance of axillary crutches like shuffling gait, dragging gait and swing gait. However walking should be trained in a gradual manner. The lower limbs are supported with appropriate orthoses and the patient is made to stand in the parallel bar. The patient is advised to do hyperextension at the hips and trunk to maintain erect posture and balance. Hyperextension of the hip locks the hip with the help of ischiofemoral ligament and thus provides stability. Once the patient is confident in standing gait training is started by instructing the patient to lift one leg and take weight on other extremity. Stepping forward is taught next and the physiotherapist progresses to walking in parallel bars. After this patient is made to walkout of the parallel bar with the help of walker. Depending on the trunk stability and confidence of the patient progression can be made to axillary crutches. Elbow crutches or canes can be given only if the upper limb musculature becomes quite strong to weight bear efficiently and within the safety limit of the patient. Even if the patient is not going to be a community walker, it is important to give him gait training so that he can achieve some independency in activities of daily living (ADL) and to maintain his self-esteem. Weight bearing on the lower limbs in erect posture also acts to slow down the process of osteoporosis and prevent tightness.

- *Use of orthosis or appliances:* Lower limb orthosis or gaiter may be used depending on the muscular status in the lower limbs.

Social and Economical Rehabilitation

The therapist should not only aim to give physical independence to the patient but should also aim to provide him with some sort of economical independency so that he feel socially acceptable. This is very important especially in younger individuals who have family members dependent on them. A group approach including Physiotherapist, Occupational therapist, Social worker and patient himself form a team and the contribution of everyone is important. Since the end user is the patient the motivation and moral of the patient should be kept high during the whole process. The patient should be provided a job he is interested in and is able to manage with his physical disability. Since the patient is a paraplegic he may be used to perform those job that involves the skill of the upper limb. Having a good trunk control will be an added asset during this stage of vocational rehabilitation. With the emergence of software technology, the employment opportunity has increased in recent years for this kind of disabled patient. Vocational training may be implemented if the patient doesn't have a particular skill necessary to have a job. Carvings, embroidery, computer jobs, and other forms of deskwork can be taught to the patient. Once the patient earns his living it will not only give him economical independence but will also keep him engaged so that he no longer keeps thinking about his impairment but focuses his attention on a much more positive aspect of life.

The overall rehabilitation of the patient depends upon his motivation, and determination along with skill, perseverance of the therapist.

SELF-ASSESSING QUESTIONS

- What are the causes of paraplegia?
- Discuss the management of paraplegia.
- Give the complication of paraplegia.
- Write a note on wheelchair management.
- Write a note on significance of home adaptation and vocational rehabilitation for paraplegia.

12

Cerebral Palsy

Cerebral palsy is a term used to describe a broad spectrum of motor disability which is non-progressive and is caused by damage to brain at or around birth. It is a disorder which develops due to damage to CNS and this damage can take place before, during, or immediately after the birth of the child. The damage won't worsen but remains constant. However the child may appear to worsen if not given proper intervention not because of an increase in lesion in the brain but just because the damaged brain is not able to cope up with the physical demand of the growing body and the increasing demand of the environment surrounding the child.

CAUSES

Antenatal Causes

Genetic causes: First or second degree consanguineous marriage.
Intrauterine virus infection: Rubella and cytomegalovirus infections which lead to severe brain damage along with associated visual and hearing problem with cataract.
Hypoglycemia: Low blood sugar for long period lead to brain damage and epilepsy. Cerebellum is more vulnerable leading to ataxia and visual problems. Infant of diabetic mothers are more prone to hypoglycemia.
Trauma to the mother.
Infection to the mother can make the baby prone to develop it.
Malnourishment of the fetus especially in case of twins.
Exposure of the mother's abdominal area to repeated X-ray radiation
Prolonged use of medications like steroids by mother.

Neonatal Causes

Prematurity: Premature babies are more prone to brain damage either due to trauma during delivery and later on due to immature respiratory and cardiovascular system. Therefore they are likely to develop hypoxia and low blood pressure also, they are more likely to develop low blood sugar, jaundice and hemorrhage because of liver immaturity.

Vascular causes: Occlusion of the internal carotid or midcerebral artery during birth can on many occasions lead to hemiplegia.

Trauma: Trauma can occur either due to disproportion, breech delivery, forceps delivery, rapid delivery, distortion of head and tearing of tentorium.

Asphyxia: It can occur by accidents and burns which could be as a result of knotted umbilical cord, cord around the neck or prolapsed cord. Multiple deliveries can cause asphyxia of the second or third infant.

Neonatal meningitis: Usually associated with severe residual brain damage.

Postnatal Causes

Delayed cry: Causes asphyxia to the brain causing CP.

Severe jaundice: Presence of high levels of bilirubin cause basal ganglia damage leading to athetoid cerebral palsy and high tone deafness.

Trauma: Fall of the body after birth

Infection: Like meningitis, or encephalitis can cause brain damage.

NORMAL DEVELOPMENT

Motor Development

Here we take into consideration dynamic movements, which are under voluntary control. Dynamic movements allow us to maintain an erect and stable posture and based on this posture we can carry-out various finer movements. The movements in supine position are not dynamic movements. For dynamic movements to take place patient should be erect without support. The movements are controlled at higher levels and by spinal cord reflex mechanism. All movements have two components, motor and sensory.

Motor developments depend upon the growth and developments of CNS, genetic factors, and environmental or external factors.

Development is a progression through which one attains maturity and is a continuous and orderly process. Stages of developments can be divided as development of the fetus and development after birth.

Maturity is the ultimate limit of anatomical and physiological changes that is genetically determined. Development is in cephalocaudal order which means proximal to distal and is true in fetus and infants. It always starts from midline to the periphery. The movements seen in infants are mass movements that do not have any rhythm or coordination and when later on the development takes place, these movements are converted to isolated movements.

When a child is born tracts are unmyelinated hence isolation or inhibition are not possible. As myelination occurs child can carry-out isolated movements. Hence neonates develop from generalized to specific behavior. It is at this stage that various primitive reflex patterns also become apparent. These primitive reflex patterns serve as a basis for motor functions throughout life.

Primitive reflex patterns: These are patterns seen in early stages of development which disappear later on or with advanced age. These reflex are essential for normal progressive motor development. There are some children who may skip some movements but these are not abnormal. However not overcoming these primitive reflex patterns at the right time should be definitely considered as abnormal. Initially lower centers such as spinal cord control these movements but later on higher centers like midbrain and cortex take control over them and dominate the lower ones thus integrating them for various voluntary functional task. Disappearance of certain primitive reflex does not mean they are abolished but means that they have been take over by stronger reflexes at higher level in the CNS.

These primitive reflexes are classified according to the level at which they are controlled. Accordingly we have four levels at which these reflexes are regulated:
1. Spinal cord
2. Brainstem
3. Midbrain
4. Cortex

There is a fifth category called *Automatic reflexes* under which we have Moro's reflex, Gallants trunk incurvatum, Landau's reflexes and Parachute reflex.

Spinal reflex
• Flexor withdrawal

- Extensor trust
- Cross extension
- Palmar grip
- Plantar grip
- Sucking reflex
- Rooting reflex
- Primitive walking.

Brainstem reflex

This consists of all the tonic reflex
- Symmetrical tonic neck reflex
- Asymmetrical tonic neck reflex
- Tonic labyrinthine reflex
- Positive and negative supporting reactions.

Midbrain level reflex

This consists of all the righting reflexes
- Optical righting
- Labyrinthine reflex
- Body on neck
- Body on body
- Neck righting reflex.

Cortical reflex

At cortical level all are equilibrium reactions, which can be in prone, supine, kneeling, sitting and standing.

Reflex Testing

This is usually done during examination of any CP cases.

Automatic Reactions

Moro's reaction

Position: Supine.

Stimulus: Either sudden loud noise like clapping.

Reaction: Sudden abduction of upper extremities with extension followed by flexion and adduction.

It is present since birth and is normal upto 3 to 4 months. If it is present beyond 6 months it is considered pathological. Absence of any of these movements in any extremity can be suggestive of LMN lesion.

Landau's reaction

Position: Ventral suspension.
Stimulus: Either active or passive extension of neck.
Response: Hyperextension of spine and lower limbs seen around 3 months of age, reaches its peak at 8 months. Beyond 10 months is pathological.

Gallants Trunk Incurvatum

Position: Ventral suspension.
Stimulus: Stroking paraspinally from twelfth rib to the iliac crest.
Reaction: Lateral flexion and curvature of trunk to the side of stimulus.

It is present at birth and normal up to 6 months. Persistence of it is seen in child who becomes athetoid. If it is more pronounced unilaterally can give rise to scoliosis. Disappearance of this reflex suggests trunk control is developing.

Parachute Reflex

Position: Child in prone position on plinth and suddenly lifted either by holding ankle or pelvis.
Response: Sudden extension of upper limb which is in order to protect head. It appears around 6 months and remains throughout life.

Spinal Level Reflex or Nociceptive Reflex

Flexor Withdrawal

Position: Supine head in neutral position and legs extended.
Stimulus: Sole of foot.
Response: Uncontrolled flexion of stimulated extremity.

This is present since birth and disappears by 2 months.

Extensor Trust

Position: Supine head neutral one leg extended and the other flexed.
Stimulus: Sole of flexed leg is given stroking.

Response: Immediate extension adduction and internal rotation of flexed leg with plantar flexion of foot.
Present at birth and integrated by 4 months.

Cross Extensor

Position: Same as extensor trust.
Stimulus: Medial aspect of extended leg.
Response: Immediate extension adduction and internal rotation of flexed leg with plantar flexion of foot.
   Present since birth and integrated by 2 months.

Plantar and Palmar Grasp

Stimulus: Press some object on palm from ulnar side.
Response: Grasping of the object on the ulnar side.
Stimulus: Press object on the plantar side of toes laterally.
Response: Clawing and clutching .
   Both these reflexes are present since birth and integrate on 10 months. Normal grasp and release cannot develop unless the palmar grip is present and normal walking cannot develop until plantar grasp is present.

Sucking and Rooting

Stimulus: Finger touching or going into child's mouth.
Response: Turning of head of child in the direction of stimulus and appears as though the child is sucking the object. Present at birth and integrates within 3 to 6 months.

Brainstem Level

Asymmetrical tonic neck reflexes
Position: Child is supine, head neutral and limbs relaxed.
Stimulus: Turning of head of child towards one side.
Response: Extension of limbs on face side and flexion of the limb on the occipital side.
   Present at 2 months of age and integrated by 4 to 6 months If ATNR is predominant then hand to mouth reaction is affected, hand coordination is affected and midline activity like rolling over doesn't develop.

Symmetrical Tonic Neck Reflex

Position: The child is in quadripedal position.

Stimulus: The head is either flexed or extended.

Response: When the head is in flexion, the upper limb gets flexed and lower limb extends, similarly when the head is extended the upper limb goes into extension and the lower limb goes into a flexed position.

This reflex is present from 4 months and should disappear by 6 months. If present after that then the child is unable to crawl. Same reflex can also be checked in sitting.

Tonic Labyrinthine Reflex

Position: Either supine or prone

Response: As the position itself is the stimulus, if the child is in supine position then there is increase in tone in the extensor group of muscles and when the child is kept in prone position then there is increase in tone in the flexor group of muscles.

This reflex is present from birth and integrates by 3 to 4 months. With the disappearance of this reflex head control will begin.

If it is present in supine then lifting of head, kicking is not possible but midline activity is possible. However if it is present in prone position then head raising and reaching over is not possible. If you put such a child in sitting position he will be sitting on the sacrum or if the head is allowed to extend there will be extension of the entire body and the child will fall backward.

Positive Supporting Reaction

Stimulus: Hold child in erect position, lift him up and bounce up and down on plinth till sole of the foot touches the plinth.

Response: Exaggerated extension of the lower limbs.

This is present at birth and disappears within 3 to 4 months.

Negative supporting reaction can be checked by holding the child in weight bearing position and suddenly lift him up. The response is sudden flexion of the lower limbs. This is present at birth and integrated by 4 months.

Midbrain Level Reflex

Optical righting reflex

Position: Hold child from armpit in a suspended position then change position of his head from side to side.

Response: Eyes will always move to same side as head.

It appears by 1 to 2 years and remains throughout one's life.

Labyrinthine Reflex

Position: Blind fold child, hold in supine position from side line.
Response: Head comes to neutral.

Seen by 2 to 3 months, reaches peak by 5 to 6 months.

Neck Righting

Position: Supine blind folded. Rotate head to one side.
Response: Body rotates to that side as a whole. Generally present at birth but a time may appear as late as 3 months.

Body on neck

Position: Supine Blind folded.
Stimulus: Rotate body to one side.
Response: Head turns in line of body. Present since 6 months and remains throughout one's life.

Body on body

Position: Blind folded.
Stimulus: Rotation of pelvis to one side..
Response: The trunk and shoulder follow direction of pelvis. It is called as segmental rolling.

These reflexes present from 6 months onward and remains throughout one's life.

Cortical Level Reflex

This consists of all the equilibrium reactions. It is usually checked on tilt board or rocking board. Look for extension of upper or lower extremities in direction of tilt (prevent any injuries).

Equilibrium reaction in supine and in prone position is present from 6 months onwards. Equilibrium reaction in quadripedal position is present from 8 months. Equilibrium in sitting starts normally from 10-12 months. Kneeling equilibrium occurs from 15 months onwards and finally equilibrium reactions in standing occur from 18 months onwards.

ABNORMAL MANIFESTATIONS

- A patient with spinal cord dominance will not be able to walk and carry out ADL and therefore he will be bedridden throughout his life. The condition gives rise to lot of contractures. Hence the treatment aims primarily at preventing secondary complication due to lack of ambulation like preventing tightness or contractures, respiratory complication, etc. need to be taken care of.
- Child with brainstem dominance will also be bedridden and unable to walk. Aim of the treatment will be similar to the above situation where all secondary complications due to lack of ambulation need to be prevented.
- Midbrain dominance children will have a relatively better prognosis. Such a child can ambulate but due to and or absent equilibrium reactions some walking aids are required.
- Cortical dominance children will have a near normal development.

NORMAL MOTOR DEVELOPMENT

Development and growth are interlinked. These are continuous process. There are two major growth spurts, one from fetal up to 6 years and the other from prepubertal up to adolescence. Growth includes physical, intellectual and emotional.

Physical growth consists of change in the size and function, Intellectual consists of skills in wise thinking and Emotional growth consists of ability to establish interpersonal bonds.

Fetal growth extends from 0 to 12 weeks during which organogenesis takes place. First trimester hazards consists of:
- Hazard of faulty implantation
- Embryonic defect
- Maternal infection.

Second trimester is relatively safe and the fetus gains about 70 percent of height and 20 percent of birth weight.

Third trimester consists of hazards such as:
- Hazard of abortion and infection
- Rapid weight gain.

The normal weight gain is about 0.4 pounds per week. At birth normal average height is about 20 + or – 2 inches. At one year it is about 30 + or – 2 inches. The body proportion also changes as child grows, the upper to lower segmental ratio at birth equals to about 1.7:1, at 6 months is 1.6:1, at 1 year is 1.5:1 and at 9 years it is 1:1.

Even in the neonatal period, 10 percent of total body weight is lost after which there is gradual weight gain by 30 gm per day. By 6 months it becomes the original body weight. By 1 year it is triple the original body weight.

Common factors affecting the normal motor development:
• Hereditary
• Sex
• Race
• Environmental, climatic and geographic factors
• Prematurity
• Congenital defects
• Inborn disorders
• Malnutrition
• Hormonal factors
• Repeated infections
• Emotional factors.

The development includes:
1. Motor development.
2. Visual development.
3. Social and adaptive development.
4. Speech.

Motor Development

1st Month: Only mass movements are seen as myelination is incomplete and spinal cord dominates. In prone position there is total head lag and flexed attitude. There is constant kicking and hands are close to the body with a tight fist.

2nd Month: If the child is put in prone position, he raises his head to 45 degrees and is able to hold for some-time.

3rd Month: Child raises head to 90 degree in prone. The fist starts opening out slowly but elbows are flexed and shoulder abducted.

4th Month: Child starts bearing some weight on arm and forearm. With this he is able to extend trunk to some extent. It you put the child from supine to sitting he will still present some amount of head lag. But in sitting he will have better head control. Trunk will be totally flexed and there will be sacral sitting. In supine there is midline activity which gives rise to beginning of coordination between 2 hands.

5th Month: Palms completely open up and there is some amount of elbow extension with shoulder extension. This goes on till 6th month. He starts bearing much more weight on his upper extremities which gives rise to better scapular fixation. Once this is developed then the child can shift himself on either extremities and reach out with other hand. Around same period if you put the child supine you will see kicking which will be more efficient with external rotation and more extension at the hip. Around the same period he starts rolling over from supine to prone and then prone to supine. Head lag totally disappears in this stage.

7th month and 8th month: Child starts sitting with support and also the sitting is more erect. If the child goes prone he will come up on extended hand and extension of trunk reaches maximum. From this time onwards the child starts crawling. During this time the child learns to sit from prone and learns to sit well without support. At little later stage which is around 9th month he will hold some object and pull to standing.

11th and 12th month: Child comes to standing and remains standing without any support around 1 year. The child can maintain standing as Landau is at its peak. Around the same time child learns to walk initially unilaterally to begin with and then bilaterally.

Next 4 to 5 months he can walk without support which is called as toddling.

Around 2 years the child achieves balanced walking

2 and half to 3 years he can run and climb up and down.

Visual Development

First 10 days: Doll's eye phenomenon.

2nd to 4th weeks: Brief eye following upto 45 degrees. Generally disregards but occasionally regards objects at 90 degrees.

8 to 10 weeks: Definite regard of rattle.

12 week=3 months: Regards more definite and can look around. Visual motor coordination is absent.

16 weeks=4 months: Visual field is 180 degrees and there is development of proper eye-hand coordination.

Social Development

1st month: The child stares at the surrounding and quietness down on hearing sounds

2nd month: Starts giving social smile. If this is lacking it indicates that the child may likely be having Mental retardation.

3rd month: The child starts recognizing people around him.

4th month: Hand regards present. It should disappear by 6th month. Persistence of this indicates the presence of mental retardation. By this month the cortical organization starts.

6th to 7th month: In supine position, great toe into mouth, which implies breaking down of total pattern. Reaching out and grasping is till with whole hand. Perception manipulation behavior is significant. Chewing should come by 7 month. Absence of this indicates MR.

8th to 9th month: The child responds to its name.

9th to 11th month: Manipulation ability improves. Pushing and poking ability comes in at this time. There is awareness of more than 1 object and therefore can combine two objects. Release is still crude. During release pincher group dominates. Idea about in and out develops.

12th to 15th month: Coordination develops and the child can make a tower of 2 cubes. Imitates himself in front of mirror, begins to point out and can even localize.

18th months: Toilet activity regulated during night. The child can make tower of 2 to 3 cubes. Idea about circles, oblique objects sets in this stage.

2 years: Ask for toilet during day. Makes a tower of 6 to 7 cubes. Plays with dolls and scribbles.

3 years: Feeds himself put on socks and buttons cloths. The child is generally independent.

Development of Speech

Speech has four components, which are: speaking, writing, hearing and reading.

1st month: Small throcking sounds. Hearing is indicated as the child quietness down on hearing sounds.

3rd to 4th month: Cooing.

4th month: Laughs aloud.

7th to 8th month: Squeals, mum-mum sounds.

9th month: Speaks monosyllables

10th month: Da-Da, mama and one word.
12th to 13th month: The vocabulary includes 2 other words. Responses to "give it to me" commands.

15th month: The vocabulary improves to 4 to 6 words. Points and localizes wants.

18th month: Can speak up to 10 words. Meaningless muttering and unintelligible speech.

2nd year: Joins 2 to 3 words, starts scribbling names and can identify 2 to 3 pictures.

3rd year: Can speak sentences, useful name and generally normal speech.

Classification of Cerebral Palsy

I. Topographical Classification

a. *Quadriplegia:* Involvement of four limbs.
   In this arms are more affected than leg.
   It is also called double hemiplegia.
b. *Diplegia:* Involvement of four limbs with leg more affected than hands.
c. *Paraplegia:* Involvement of both legs only.
d. *Triplegia:* Involvement of three limbs.
e. *Hemiplegia:* Involvement of one side of body.
f. *Monoplegia:* One limbs affected

II. According to Types

a. Spastic
b. Athetoid
c. Ataxic
d. Mixed.

TYPES OF CEREBRAL PALSY

Basically cerebral palsy children manifest in three common ways spastic, athetoid, and ataxic.

Spasticity seen in cerebral palsy is usually clasp knife that may change with change in position, which means that spasticity, may vary from supine to prone. In supine we see increase in extensor tone and in prone position we see increase in flexor. The tone also varies with position of head and neck. This is as a result of tonic neck reflexes and labyrinthine reflexes. Along with hypertonia there will be increase in tendon jerks, clonus in ankle and sometimes in patella and wrist. Babinski sign is positive. Voluntary control in these children is always affected and they might find difficulty in initiating the movement or difficulty may be felt during different parts of range and very often a movement is performed in an abnormal manner.

For instance, when a normal person is walking there is flexion, adduction and external rotation. On the contrary, in spastic we see extensions, adduction and internal rotation. This pattern is called *Scissoring*. Whenever the child attempts a particular movement isolation of the movement is lacking and instead the child has *Mass Movement Pattern*. Moreover there is cocontraction due to absence of reciprocal inhibition. These children also show certain abnormal postures. These postures are as a result of spastic muscle groups, which become tight and are usually associated with antigravity muscles. If these patterns of muscles are allowed to persist they lead to contractures and deformities (Fig. 12.1 Plate 6). Apart from this disability the child also has low IQ leaving some exceptional cases, visual problems, problems of perception, epilepsy (which results from instability of cells due to hypochromatolysis.

Athetoid cerebral palsy children exhibits slow, purposeless, wormlike, involuntary movements which flow into each other. It occurs due to basal ganglia damage commonly seen in children who suffers from an attack of jaundice following birth. They may follow abnormal pattern. Very often these involuntary movements are present at rest and increase with excitement, fear and effort. Hence if such a child attempts to carry-out any movement athetosis increases. Voluntary movements are possible but they lack coordination and finer movements are also lacking. There is always initial delay. The tone in these children generally fluctuates and very often there is dystonia which is a twisting type of movements that is constantly occurring and along with this sometimes there can be sudden flexor or extensor spasm. The other feature of the child is very high Intelligent quotient (IQ) which is a positive factor. The patient has hearing problem due to kernicterus. Also they may show emotional lability, which manifests as fluctuating moods. The athetoid CP have extrovert personality, dysarthria and paralysis of gaze.

Ataxia in cerebral palsy occurs due to cerebellar damage. Both balance and coordination is affected. Proximal fixation of head, shoulder girdle, trunk and pelvic girdle is poor. Lack of balance is compensated by excessive balance saving reaction of the upper limbs. Voluntary movements are clumsy and dissymmetric. They usually have hypotonia unless they are associated with spasticity as seen in mixed type of cerebral palsy.

Also ataxic cerebral palsy children have nystagmus, diadokokinesia, dysarthria, intentional tremors and tendon jerks are pendular. The IQ is low; there is a visual and hearing problem, perceptual difficulties but however it is very rare to see a pure ataxic cerebral palsy.

Home Treatment

Family involvement in the treatment of a cerebral palsy child is important. As the time given for the child is limited with each treatment session comprising of anywhere between 20 minutes to 45 minutes which may prove to be inadequate when it comes to stimulate the resources available for the child rehabilitation. Hence the family members should try to work in association with the therapist to provide maximum outcome of rehabilitation.

Parental and Family Education

Teaching them about the condition: Very often the parents are not told about the condition of the child in a frank manner. Especially in Indian condition where most of the children are from rural community, the therapist finds it difficult to make the parents aware of the child's condition in appropriate manner. Many times on being told the truth, the parents rejects the counseling or get depressed by taking the whole issue to a strong negative sense. Hence parents should be counselled about the condition without letting them get depressed and also told how much they can contribute in make the child's life worth living. The attitude and mannerism of the therapist should be practical, compassionate and convincing so as to make the parental education a successful one. Learning about CP will give the parents foundation in order to provide best help to their child. Also the parents should be encouraged to share what they have learned with other family members. Getting the parents of the child in contact with the parents of other cerebral palsy child who is recovering will definitely encourage the parents and keep them in positive frame of mind.

Providing appropriate education to the child: A cerebral palsy child if has a good IQ should be encouraged to pursue normal education. Infact the government has various policies and reservation to provide education to such disabled children. The family members should find out all such provision available and give the best education to the child. In case a child is not able to manage the conventional education in a successful manner then vocational training may be initiated with the help of social organization to help the child learn new skill, which may develop a sense of independency and responsibility in them. Special school for children with low IQ is available at many parts of our country.

The parents should work with teachers and school officials: The parents of the cerebral palsy children should be told to work with the child's teachers, school administrators, special learning consultants, and school boards to develop the best educational plan for their child. A cooperative team approach helps the child realize his or her potential.

*Provide psychological and emotional support :*As children grow he or she becomes more aware of their physical impairments and hence may get frustrated at times. It is necessary for the family members to allow them to talk about their feelings and how they feel they are being treated. Some children may fail to open up their feelings with the family members and hence may need the intervention of the therapist even in this matter. The children should be always kept happy and should be made to feel that they are an integral part of the family. The parents should treat the disabled child in par with other siblings. Too much of attention or too much of neglect both can have adverse effect on the child's psychology.

The parents should take care of themselves: The parents in an attempt to raise a physically challenged child should never ignore their priorities as that may end up having a negative influence on them which eventually can make them feel isolated from the rest of the world. Hence they should be advised to take proper rest, eat well, exercise, lead a social life and should learn different ways to cope with the challenges of raising a child with CP. The parents will only be better equipped to help their child when they have good physical energy, emotional strength and financial support.

Developing a strong bond: The entire family is affected when one member has CP. Hence motivating each other is very important. You can help prevent other children from developing unrealistic fears and concerns, feeling left out, or becoming overwhelmed. One should remember every-one in this life has some concern or other it is only the magnitude that differs, hence even in this situation the family should stay united and learn to be happy.

Helping the CP Child with Activities of Daily Living

Each person with CP has unique strengths and areas of difficulty. However, most people with CP need some level of help in the following areas:
- Feeding
- Toilet activities
- Bathing
- Combing hair
- Dressing
- Dental hygiene
- Physical security.

Encouraging the Child for Independence

Parents and other caregivers can help children with CP develop to their highest potential. One of the most important things is to help them learn to do as much for themselves as they can. Many a times parents over protect the child or show so much concern which will make them over dependent on the parents thus inhibiting them to explore their potential to perform various task

Parents must also understand that they will need to bring about some change in their own routines as their child with CP grows. For instance, parents may not be able to continue caring for a severely affected child who is growing tall and heavy. Parents also need to plan ahead for the time when their grown child with CP is not under their care.

Medical Management

Medications may be necessary to control some of the symptoms of cerebral palsy. For example if the spasticity is very severe physiotherapy intervention may be difficult hence attempts should be made to keep the symptoms under control although temporarily so that during this time effective physiotherapy program may be implemented.

Common medicines used are antispasmodics. They relax tight muscles and reduce muscle spasms. Most antispasmodics are taken orally and include:
- Diazepam (such as Valium)
- Baclofen (Lioresal)
- Dantrolene sodium (Dantrium).

Intramuscular muscle relaxants are occasionally used to relax muscles and reduce spasms. They typically remain effective for about 3 to 6 months and include:
- Phenol or alcohol "washes."
- Botox or Botulin toxins.

In case the cerebral palsy child gets epileptic seizures then antiepileptic medicines are tried which can be:
- Phenytoin (Dilantin)
- Carbamazepine (Tegretol)
- Valproate (Depakene, Depakote)
- Phenobarbital.

Dystonic CP or cerebral palsy with involuntary movements may need anticholinergic drugs like:
- Trihexyphenidyl hydrochloride (Artane)
- Benztropine methylate (Cogentin)
- Carbidopa-levodopa (Sinemet)
- Procyclidine hydrochloride (Kemadrin)
- Glycopyrrolate (Robinul)

Physical Therapy

Physical therapy is one of the most important treatments for CP that usually begins soon after being diagnosed and often continues throughout life. Some people with CP may begin physical therapy before being diagnosed, depending on their symptoms.

Special devices and equipment are needed for some people with CP to help them with specific problems. For example:
- A child who develops uneven leg length may need to wear special shoes with a higher sole and heel on the shorter leg.
- Some people who are not able to walk alone may need to use canes, crutches, walkers, or wheelchairs.

Principles of Treatment

- Careful assessment and recording of the child should be an ongoing process and not an isolated one
- Realistically plan and measures should be derived from the assessment
- Early treatment should be incorporated into the daily management of the child
- Repetition and reinforcement are essential for learning and establishing of modified motor pattern.
- Maximize sensory motor experiences
- Involvement of the child as an active participant
- Motivation of the child should be kept high throughout the course of treatment
- The treatment of the child is a team work and the therapist should involve the family members in the treatment of the child
- There should be adequate consideration for developmental training
- The abnormal tone should be modified so as to facilitate development of function
- The therapist should try to use adequate afferent stimuli
- All the purposeful active movements should be facilitated
- Secondary impairment like contractures and deformity should be kept to the minimum
- It is essential to give functional independence which may be with or without compensation.

HISTORICAL BACKGROUND OF TREATMENT

Earlier various efforts were used to treat cerebral palsy children. All these treatment approaches had varied principles and showed different insight into the conditions. These were helpful to some extent but could not be called as the complete rehabilitation program which focussed on all the aspect of development in the cerebral palsy child. However before going into various advanced and present day management of cerebral palsy child it is necessary to know about the various foundation which over a period of time has channelized the development of present approaches towards handling a cerebral palsy child.

Phelps Technique

He used various exercise modalities like massage, passive movements, active assisted movements, and condition motion using basic PNF pattern to get the desired response. There were adequate period of rest and use of braces to correct deformity.

PNF or Proprioceptive Neuromuscular Facilitation

This technique described by Knott and Voss used the sensation from the proprioceptors in the joint and muscles to get desired motor output. Training of functional pattern was the key of this approach.

Brunstrom's Approach

Although his approach was primarily used for treatment for adult hemiplegia. It definitely has some influence on cerebral palsy management. In this technique initially the primitive reflexes and synergistic movement patterns were evoked reflexly to develop some tone in the muscle and later on volitional movement were trained along the same lines.

Roods Approach

The principles of Roods technique is using cutaneous afferents to get the desired motor response through muscle afferents. Various sensations on the skin used, for instance gentle stroking was supposed to have relaxatory effect on the muscles there by used to inhibit spastic muscles. On the other hand brisk stroking, tapping, quick ice, etc. has been found to develop tone in the muscles hence can be used for cases like flaccidity.

Temple Fay

Fay suggests that human ontogenic development is based on phylogenetic development in evolution of species and hence he taught the child to move according to development sequence.

Doman and Delacato

This system described by Glen Doman and Carl Delacato includes the basic principles postulated by fay and believed that by highly systematic movements and sensory input, the undamaged brain cells can be stimulated resulting in sensory and motor development.

Vojta's Technique

This approach was given by Paslav Voyta used afferent sensory stimulating through touch, stretch and pressure for facilitation of movement. Trigger points were used to reflexly stimulate creeping, rolling or crawling activities.

Collis Technique

Erene Collis postulated various trends like early treatment, management throughout the day and inclusion of various activities of daily living like dressing, feeding toileting and washing to be included in the treatment program. Collis also believed in strict developmental order.

Conductive Education

This concept was developed by Prof. Peto which was more educational rather than medical. It consists of three central components like task series, rhythmical intensions and daily routines through group activities.

Bobath Approach

This concept was developed by Dr. K. Bobath is based on Neurodevelopmental techniques and it views development as dynamic, sequential, cephalocaudal, proximal distal, automatic before conscious, responsive and lastly adaptive. Bobath believed in inhibiting the primitive reflex pattern using reflex inhibiting techniques and encouraged promoting movements in normal pattern as well as combination.

INTEGRATED APPROACH FOR CP

The latest and most effective way of treating cerebral palsy children comprise of an integrated approach. The common physiotherapy management of CP is based upon the following guidelines

- *Developing rapport with parents and patients:* Developing rapport with patient is extremely important as any goal will be difficult to achieve without the cooperation of the patient and the relatives. The patient has to be motivated regularly to gain confidence. Only when the motivation level of the patient is very high will the child cooperate in the treatment session. The goal set for the patient should be challenging but at the same time achievable. The therapist should avoid false appreciation. The therapist should initially give maximum support and cooperation. Good feedback of the therapist is essential in the initial stages, however once the child learns various tasks the therapist support goes on decreasing. The therapist should try and understand the situation and circumstances of the parents. She should try to gain their confidence and keep their motivation level high. As the treatment of a CP child is whole day process and not necessarily restricted to the session in the clinic the support of the family members especially the parents is very high. The therapy should be carried over at home so that the child practises it.

- *Normalizing tone of the muscles:* For cases with hypotonicity slow passive movements, sustained stretch, cryotherapy over the muscle for 15 to 20 minutes, stimulation of antagonist movement and vibrations are used. On the contrary, for cases with hypotonicity weight bearing, joint compression, rhythmic stabilization, vibrations, cryotherapy in brisk manner and tapping can be used.

- *Stretching and mobility:* The muscles should be maintained at the appropriate physiological length for normal muscle control and normal postural adjustments. In CP because of delay or absence of normal movement muscles are usually in a shortened position hence stretching of the muscles is essential to increase the neuromuscular control. Length of the muscles should be maintained not only through stretching but also through various functional activities. Thus home exercises and activities are very important in addition to the therapy at the PT clinic.

- *Developing postural reaction:* Postural adjustments are essential if the child is to move freely and to adjust to various environmental demands rapidly. Motor milestones can be best achieved by good postural reactions. Postural reactions consists of righting reactions, protective extension and equilibrium reactions. Initially children first develop righting reactions. Righting reactions allow the child to orient his head in space so that the eyes and mouth are horizontal regardless of the position of the body. It also helps in maintaining the proper alignment of the head with respect to the body and *vice versa*. Once righting reaction develop in a particular position protective extension comes up. Lastly equilibrium reaction emerge which helps the patient to counteract the opposing force and enable them to maintain balance. These reactions are best developed by various exercises on vestibular ball and tilt board (Figs 12.2 and 12.3, Plate 6).

- *Sensory integration:* Sensory integration is the ability to recognize various sensations, organize them so that they can be used to perform various activities. The various functional activities incorporating different objects, sizes, color, textures, weight can be given in the therapy.
- *Oromotor control training:* Oromotor function depends on good head control. Common oromotor problems are: drooling, problems in sucking, swallowing, body movements associated with speech, jaw, hyper or hyposensitivity and inadequate tongue movements. Hence the therapy should consists of good neck control, developing good trunk control, use of brush to decrease drooling.

Occupational therapy: Child helps adapt to their limitations and live as independently as possible.

Speech therapy helps control the mouth muscles. This therapy can be of great benefit to children with speech or eating problems. Speech therapy often starts before the child begins school and continues throughout the school years.

Nutritional counseling may help when dietary needs are not met because of problems with eating certain foods.

Biofeedback may be useful as part of physical therapy or on its own. During a biofeedback session, people with CP learn how to control their affected muscles. Some people learn ways to reduce muscle tension with this technique. Biofeedback does not help everyone with CP.

Both *massage therapy* and *hatha yoga* benefit some people with CP by helping them relax tense muscles, strengthen muscles, and keep joints flexible. Hatha yoga breathing exercises help some people relax and may prevent lung infections.

SELF-ASSESSING QUESTIONS

- What is cerebral palsy? Give the various causes for the same.
- What are the causes of cerebral palsy and give the importance of early detection of cerebral palsy?
- Principles of neurodevelopmental approaches.
- Describe various reflexes at brainstem level, midbrain level, spinal cord level.
- Explain parental education on child handling in cerebral palsy
- Describe management of cerebral palsy child.
- Rationale for Vojta's technique.
- What are the different types of cerebral palsy?

13

Poliomyelitis

Poliomyelitis is an infectious disease, epidemic and endemic in nature throughout the world. It is basically a virus infection of nerve cells in the anterior gray matter (anterior horn cells of the spinal cord), or cranial nerve nuclei in the brainstem leading in many cases to temporary or permanent paralysis of the muscles that they activate. It is a disease which occurs exclusively in humans. It is more common in Asian and African countries.

CAUSE

It is caused by infection with a virus of which at least three types have been identified as type I (Brunhilde), type II (Lanchi) and type III (Leon).

Mode of Transmission of the Virus

Poliomyelitis appears to spread mainly by fecal contamination (orofecal) route in countries where hygiene is poor and by droplet infection where the sanitation is good. The poliovirus is one of the many enteroviruses that colonize in the GIT.

Incubation Period of Virus

It varies from 3 to 30 days while 7 to 14 days is the most common interval between infection and the clinical illness. This incubation period decreases on provocation like injection pricks, stenosis, physical activities, massage or minor operation. In infants below six months the involvement may be transplacentally transmitted if the maternal immunity is very low.

PATHOLOGY

The disease occurs in 3 stages.

Alimentary Stage

After gaining access to the body through the nasopharynx or the GIT, the virus multiplies in the epithelial cells of the intestinal mucosa.

Viremic Stage

The virus spreads into the blood stream and after a sort of conflict between the virus and the antibodies, in case the virus turns victorious then it leads to the third stage.

Neural Stage

The virus finds its way to the anterior horn cells of the spinal cord and some times to nerve cells in the brainstem. According to the virulence of the infection the cells may escape serious harm or they may be damaged or killed. If cells are damaged there is paralysis of the corresponding muscles but recovery is possible. However if the cells are killed then the paralysis is permanent.

CLINICAL FEATURES

The course of the disease is divided into four different stages and each with its own clinicopathological picture and varied treatment.

Prodromal Stage or Pre-Paralytic Stage

It is nonspecific and mimics any viral infection. The illness is usually of vague and variable duration. It may last from a few hours to a few days and 1 to 3 days is the usual duration. It may be severe or so mild as to pass unnoticed. It is usually but not always followed by an asymptomatic stage before the onset of the paralysis. Many patients never progress beyond this stage and are only diagnosed by the laboratory findings of the poliovirus in the throat or the stools. The importance of this stage is that exercise, injections or operations may precipitate severe paralysis in the limbs exercised or traumatized.

Signs and Symptoms

The most common ones are headache, sore throat, malaise, slight cough, diarrhea or constipation, backache, joint pains, pyrexia of variable duration and severity, mild neck stiffness and irritability.

Many other symptoms may occur and the only way to deal with the problem is to regard all children with the above symptoms as suspect during an epidemic.

Treatment

When the facility allows all the suspects should be put to bed and rested if possible. This is of course completely impracticable in many developing countries. The only practical measures which can be taken in suspects in economically poor countries is to stop the playing of games and other such manual work if possible. Chances of infection should be avoided especially the most severe general infections. Performance of tonsillectomies and other such non-emergency surgery should be discouraged during the peak of an epidemic of polio.

The nasopharyngeal secretions and feces are highly infective at this stage of illness and children with suspected infections should be isolated if possible particularly from other children and babies. An additional booster dose may be given to the affected and unaffected children which will also act as an added protection.

Acute Stage

If the infection does not resolve in the prodromal stage it enters the acute stage which is the early stage of paralysis. Here most of the signs and symptoms remains similar to the prodromal stage but are more pronounced especially the following:
- Fever—variable in both duration and severity
- Diarrhea, nausea and vomiting
- Irritability
- Limb and joint pains — This is due to painful surrounding muscles. There is never any swelling or redness of joints. This is an important differentiating point from acute arthritis
- Muscle tenderness is the most important sign seen in this stage.

To test this press the calf muscles when the child is quiet. If he cries it means he has tenderness. The child prefers a sleeping position and can not tolerate change of position. He can have upper respiratory tract infection also.

Duration: 3 to 6 weeks from the onset of Poliomyelitis.

Treatment

Rest: The child should not be over handled. Over handling of the children during this stage will definitely aggravate the condition and may increase the muscle damage. All the physical activity should be discouraged at this stage. Minimal handling of the child will prevent movement to the lumbar spine and thereby help in decreasing the chances of aggravation of symptoms. Infact, the therapist should not call the patient daily on OPD basis for treatment. Isolation: The affected child should be isolated and prevented from mingling with other children in the house or from the surrounding. This is necessary to protect the other children from contacting the infection because stools, urine and droplets are highly contaminated and contagious.

Booster dose: The other children in the house should be given booster dose of the vaccination.

Nutrition: The affected children should be given diet rich in protein.

Correct handling technique: The parents of the child should be taught correct handling technique that will prevent any further damage to the neural structures. The child should not be lifted by one hand and while carrying the child they should be held in front and preferably with the hip in extension without any abduction.

Splintage and correct positioning: Splintage given so that the lower limb can be immobilized so as to prevent any further damage to the muscles. Moreover giving a splint also reduces the pain arising from the muscles by immobilizing them and offering support. Splinting in this stage also prevents the muscles from going into contractures.

Sister Kenny's bath: It is a form of moist heat. Here a towel is dipped in hot water and wringed. Then it is placed on the limbs and lumbar spine of the patient. This is a form of wet, moist heat that helps to resolve inflammation to some extent. Massage should not be given as it may cause more damage due to which the patient may not be able to walk later on. Any form of trauma to the muscles should be avoided.

MMT: Immediately after the muscular pain gets reduced and the patient comes out of the initial stages of inflammation, manual muscle charting should be done to know the extent of weakness or paralysis.

Gentle passive movement: The parents of the child should be shown to do gentle passive movement at least 2 to 3 times per day mainly to keep the muscle and joint flexible as well as to improve circulation to the limbs. This depends on the tolerance of the patient and should not be given when the muscles are painful or tender.

Convalescent Stage

This is the stage where there is true or actual paralysis. The duration of this stage is 3 months. Here the sign and symptoms are very variable in both duration and severity. The extent and distribution of the lesion vary widely from case to case. Thus the effects may lead to paralysis which may take on one of these forms:
1. Spinal
2. Bulbar
3. Spinobulbar/bulbospinal
4. Postencephalitic type of paralysis. However the most common is the spinal type. The most fatal one is the encephalitic type of paralysis.

Spinal Type

Here the anterior horn cells are affected with resulting paralysis of a lower motor neuron type with asymmetrical flaccid paralysis and normal sensation.

The muscles affected depend on which anterior horn cells of spinal cord is involved but the paralysis tends to affects certain muscles more commonly than other muscles. The lower limb muscles are more often involved than the upper limb muscles. Moreover the involvement of muscles is very asymmetrical and this offers a valuable distinguishing factor while differentiating polio from Guillain-Barré syndrome. Due to gross muscular imbalance as a result of such paralysis contractures are liable to occur. Contractures eventually leads to deformity which are particularly seen in the lower limbs where the flexors of the hip, knee and ankle are often less paralyzed than the extensors. Flexion contractures of the hip, knee and equines deformity of the ankle are therefore common sequel.

Bulbar Type

The most important sign of bulbar paralysis is the inability to swallow due to pharyngeal paralysis. The patient chokes on both solid and liquid food and cannot swallow his own saliva. In addition the patient cannot cough properly due to paralysis of larynx. He also has difficulty in speaking due to paralysis of the palate. The respiratory muscles (intercoastals and diaphragmatic) or swallowing muscles or both are affected and thus the patient requires urgent treatment to save his life in the form of ventilatory support for respiration and intubation with Ryle's tube for feeding.

The early signs of respiratory involvement includes breathlessness, a feeling of suffocation, slight cyanosis and the use of sternomastoids, alae nasae as well as other accessory muscles of respiration.

Spinobulbar

In this type there is combination of both spinal and bulbar type of polio. Some patients may present with predominant spinal presentation and less bulbar in which case it is called as spinobulbar. Some patients may have more bulbar sings and less spinal sings in which case it is called as bulbospinal type.

Postencephalitic

This is rare and is usually associated with bulbar paralysis. Mental disturbance and even coma may occur. There is nearly always paralysis of the facial muscles. Symptoms similar to meningitis like headache, vomiting, neck stiffness, etc. may be seen.

In addition there may be transient involvement of the bladder with urinary retention that always improves. The degree of initial paralysis bears little relation to the final degree of recovery.

Treatment

Continuous splintage: Above knee splint or even L splint may be given to prevent knee flexion and equines deformity. Below knee splint may be sufficient if the patient has a tendency to develop equines deformity. Weakness of the abdominal muscles especially patchy type may cause protrusion of the organ from the weaker spot due to lack of proper abdominal support hence the patient may be given abdominal corset. The abdominal corset is like a lumbar corset but in the absence of it even a towel can be wrapped tightly around the abdomen. In case of patchy abdominal paralysis which leads to abdominal hernia, a cardboard piece is placed over that area and then the towel is tied. This gives better stabilization and counter pressure. This should be loosened while feeding and should not interfere with respiration. Chest PT can be given with the corset on as it gives a good intra-abdominal pressures.

Muscle charting: It is important to assess all the muscle groups as soon as the tenderness in the muscles will allow which usually is after 3 to 4 weeks after the onset of paralysis. The degree of recovery should then be assessed at succeeding attendance, which means that MMT should be done every week or at least alternate week.

Some-times one set of MMT needs to be done in 2 to 3 sittings as in children it is difficult to do it in a single sitting. More-over one should not induce fatigue to the patient as it may interfere with the treatment and prognosis of the condition. Thus an appropriate idea as to the final degree of recovery and the necessity for calliperization can be known at 3 months approximately.

Positioning: Patient's relatives should be told not to carry the child in Indian position as this tends to increase the IT band contractures. Also while sleeping the child should be kept prone preferably to avoid hip flexion contractures. Paralyzed arms are best supported on pillows with slight degree of abduction. In the upper limbs deltoid is the most common muscle to get paralyzed hence the child should never be pulled up holding his hands as this may lead to shoulder subluxation due to tendency of head of humerus to come down due to gravity. Shoulder rolls in the form of towel rolled and kept under the axilla helps to prevent shoulder subluxation as it offers an upward pressure. This should be given for at least 3 months. It can also be tied all round. This has to be maintained throughout even when the child is sleeping or being carried around.

Changing the position: A severely paralyzed patient should be turned every 2 to 4 hours day and night to prevent bed sores from developing and also to keep the skin dry.

Stretching of contractures: The tight and contracted soft tissue should be gently but consistently stretched to prevent the chances of gross deformity. The principal contractures are IT band and ankle equines.

If the tendo Achilles is weak with grade either 0 or 1 then while stretching it out excessive stretch should be avoided, as there is more anterior gliding of tibia which could lead to calcaneal deformity. Therefore it should be stretched only to neutral position. IT band contracture needs full stretching normally but in cases where there is gluteus medius weakness, full stretching of IT band will further weaken the gluteus medius due to excessive stretch and will lead to or exaggerated Trendelenburg lurch. Thus in cases where there is a gluteus medius weakness a decision has to be made whether to stretch it fully or to stretch it only to neutral.

Stimulation and facilitation technique: If the patient can tolerate then IG stimulation may be given to maintain the muscular property so that it facilitates improvement in the next stage. Even technique like stroking briskly the affected muscles will help in facilitation.

Stage of Recovery

This stage is also called a late convalescent stage. This stage extends up to almost 2 years. Thus the muscles in polio patient can be strengthened to their maximum capacity up to 2 years after this it won't be possible to activate any paralyzed muscles. However the already active muscle may show some improvement even after 2 years due to some positive changes in the muscular structure. Infact whatever improvement in muscle power the patient's receives after this time limit could be primarily due to hypertrophy of the muscle fibers in the recovering muscles. Before 2 years time if any muscle is seen to regaining the power, it must be exercised quite skill fully to achieve maximum rehabilitation output. Infact it is always better if the strengthening program is initially gently and later on vigorous. Various form of strengthening techniques may be used which could be as follows:

1. Sensory integration: Here various sensory stimuli are used to get the motor response. This technique is used very much in the children who are below the comprehending or understanding age group.
2. If the patient can understand then resisted exercises with the help of springs and pulleys are given.
3. Hydrotherapy and suspension therapy.
4. PNT techniques like timing for emphasize which uses the over flow principles are found to be very effective.
5. Play therapy: Involving the children in some out door games also helps in improving the strength of upper limb and lower limb. The game selected should be specific with respect to the muscle that needs to be strengthened. As games forms a type of recreational activity children usually cooperate better. However

this should be done with lot of caution to prevent any injury to the child.

6. Mat exercises: These exercises can be given to bring about an over all improvement in the coordination, functional activities, etc. Weight bearing exercises should be taught at the right time because if the child does not weight bear at the right age then various changes occurs in the bone due to interference with the absorption of important minerals by the bone. For instance, the acetabulum tends to become shallow due to lack of weight bearing pressure.

As a particular milestone age is reached and if the child is unable to do then he must be passively put in that position. With repetition the CNS learns that particular activity.

If the patient can't stand he should be made to do so with some external support like splints or parallel bars, etc. so that later when he undergoes calliperization and gait training it is easy for him because he has already experienced the erect posture and force of gravity.

Stage of Residual Paralysis

Paralysis or weakness persisting after 2 years is permanent. Whatever improvement may be seen could be attributed to the increase in the size of the available muscle fibers or muscles. The extent of residual paralysis ranges between mild insignificant local weakness to almost gross paralysis of the trunk and limbs musculature giving rise to severe disability and functional dependency. Weakness and wasting of the muscle causes impaired growth of the bone which gets shortened. Moreover, gross muscular imbalance coupled with limb length discrepancy causes deformity of the trunk and the limbs.

Treatment

Once the patient reaches the stage of PPRP (Post polio residual palsy), then his intervention is like any other orthopedic cases as the problem is more mechanical than neurological. Usually the patient may be given a combination of stretching, strengthening and calliperization. Serial casting in combination with exercises have proved to be very effective in correcting deformity. Sometimes correcting the deformity suddenly can grossly interfere with the compensatory mechanisms that has given the patient functional independency in which case a tailor-made calliper can be given to accommodate the deformity and at the same time giving support to prevent any chances of mechanical stress from falling on the joint. Also a tailor-made calliper can also prevent the deformity from aggravating.

However in case conservative mode of treatment fail to correct a deformity then the patient may be referred for surgical intervention which may involve either soft tissue release or lengthening, osteotomies, etc. Tendon transfers may be done in case there is availability of good donor muscles without compromising on the balance on that side. Arthrodesis is other surgery which is preferred especially around the ankle in case there are severe instability making weight bearing difficult.

Common Problems Encountered by Polio Patients

Muscle weakness: Because the anterior horn cells are involved there is a lower motor neuron type of paralysis. There is no sensory loss. Lower limbs are more affected than upper limbs. Abdominal may or may not be affected and can rarely be affected without affection of the upper limb or lower limbs. In the lower limb most commonly affected muscle is the *Tibialis anterior*. Most of the time it could be the only muscle involved the patient. Infact if on MMT, tibialis anterior is graded is 3 or more then the diagnosis of polio is doubtful. Besides it could also have been that the action of the weak tibialis anterior is substituted by Extensor hallucis longus due to closer proximity. Therefore, careful grading must be done. Other muscles which are also prone to be affected are Quadriceps, Gluteus maximus, Gluteus medius. In the upper limb biceps, triceps or deltoid are the most common muscles. However there can be involvement of other muscles as well.

Abdominal: In a child if the abdominal muscles are weak, then when he cries the organs may protrude through the weaker part in the abdominal region creating a bulge which goes back once the child stops crying. This is because of the increase in the intra-abdominal pressure that cannot be counteracted by the weak abdominus.

Bony changes: Most common bony changes is:

Shortening: Shortening of the bones occurs due to lack of muscle pull on them. These can be Shortening of the limb which is not proportionate or directly related to muscle involvement. The reason for this is not known however it is thought that the poliovirus directly affects the bone and causes shortening.

Osteoporosis: It is an indirect effect of polio and it is due to,
a. Lack of muscle contraction
b. Immobilization
c. Lack of weight bearing hence more prone to fractures.

Therefore over stretching of deformities must be prevented or there may be fractures, e.g. during stretching of the tendo Achilles, there may be fracture of shaft tibia. Similarly on stretching the IT bands there may be fracture neck femur distal to the point of support.

Deformities: The initial cause of deformities in poliomyelitis appears to be muscle spasm followed by interstitial fibrosis and collagen deposition in paretic muscle groups. This may lead to severe deformities as early as a month after the onset of paralysis. The exact cause of muscle spasm is unknown but basically it appears to be due to involuntary contraction of surviving fibers in partially paralyzed muscles.

Although the spasm of muscles is important in acute polio, the growth of the limb is the most important factors in the progress of all deformities in chronic polio. This is why deformities are always more worse in children than in the adult or in the adolescence. Deformities are always seen in combinations and are not necessarily be related to muscle weakness. In short, muscle imbalance as a result of weakness and tightness leads to contractures and deformity. The most common muscles that causes deformities due to contractures are:
a. IT band contractures that causes flexion, abduction and external rotation at hip with knee flexion and genu valgus.
b. TA contracture causes equines deformity at the ankle which in turn causes the hip and knee to go into flexion as a result of apparent lengthening of the limb (Figs 13.1 and 13.2, Plate 7).

SELF-ASSESSING QUESTIONS

Long and Short Essay

- Explain stage wise management of poliomyelitis.
- Explain the clinical feature of the various stages in polio.

- What are the various stages of poliomyelitis? Give the stage wise management for the same.
- Describe the common problems encountered by a polio child.
- Give an assessment protocol for PPRP and give the management in this stage.
- What are the principles behind recovery seen in polio patient?

Short Answers

- Name the viruses causing polio.
- Name common contractures in polio child.
- List the symptoms in prodromal stage of polio.
- What are the causes of bone shortening in polio.
- Define poliomyelitis.

14

Electrophysiology

EMG

EMG is a diagnostic and therapeutic procedure which involves detecting muscle activity in the form of potentials, amplifying these signals and displaying them on the screen for study and treatment purposes.

EMG helps in testing the efficiency of the lower motor neuron by giving information about the disturbance in activity. It is useful in identifying muscular disorder, problems pertaining to the peripheral nerves and even the anterior horn cell. EMG testing needs active cooperation from the patient. It may not be performed in unconscious patients, mentally retarded patients and even in infants. Earlier days EMG was used mainly as investigations but with the availability of integrated EMG its has become an effective mode of giving feedback to the patient which in turns stimulates the patient to either facilitate the feedback or inhibit it based upon the clinical requirement.

For EMG recording one can use either a needle or surface electrode. Both these electrode have their own advantages and disadvantages. Needle electrode helps in precise sampling of the muscles required including deeper and smaller muscles without having interference from other muscles. On the contrary the disadvantage of needle electrode is that it needs to be given with utmost care to prevent the chances of infection, maintenance becomes expensive as the electrodes are disposable once which has to be changed for all patient. Also needle electrode demands greater skill from the therapist. It is invasive and hence painful.

Surface electrode on the other hand being non-invasive doesn't carry any chances of infection. It is very easy to use and doesn't cause pain to the patient. However the disadvantage of surface electrode is that deep and small muscles cannot be studied. Skin and subcutaneous tissue's interference cannot be overcome.

Routine EMG recordings are done in three stages:
1. At rest
2. Activity during mild voluntary efforts
3. Activity during maximum voluntary efforts

At rest, normally there is no activity. However if the needle electrode happens to be in the motor end plate area then the patient may exhibit end plate activity. End plate activity are of two types–end plate spike and end plate noise. Both these activity are miniature end plate potential which appear very small in amplitude. End plate noise also has a characteristic sound on the loud speaker which is similar to the sound of sea shell held to the ear. To differentiate this normal end plate activity from abnormal spontaneous activity which is also produced at rest one should reposition the needle to confirm. On repositioning if this activity at rest are not reproduced then it is normal but if they are reproduced then it may indicate the presence of spontaneous activity which is abnormal.

On mild voluntary efforts few motor unit in the recording muscles fire and this firing is displayed on the screen as motor unit potentials. These potentials are described based on the following important parameters:

Amplitude

Amplitude is measured from the positive peak to the negative peak. It indicates the total height of the potential. The amplitude of a motor unit potential is dependent on the fiber density of the motor unit. Also only those fiber which lie within the pick up area of the electrode determine the height of the potential. It is very difficult to standardize a particular range as amplitude for any given number due to various anatomical differences based upon the sex, height, weight, occupation and lifestyle of individual. However in general the amplitude ranges from anywhere between 100 microvolts to few millivolts.

Duration

The duration of the potential is measured from initial take off the potential to its return to the base line. Unlike the amplitude which depends upon the fiber density. The duration of the potential is determined by the motor unit territory, hence not only the muscle fiber near the tip of the electrode contribute but even the muscle fiber that is situated at the distance from the recording electrode but belonging to the same motor unit also contributes towards the duration of that motor unit potential. The normal duration range between 10 to 15 milliseconds.

Rise Time

The rise time is the time taken by the motor unit potential to travel from the positive peak to the negative peak. It is an indicator of the synchronicity in the firing of the muscle fiber belonging to a particular motor unit. The normal rise time is about 500 micro-seconds.

Phases

It is that part of the wave form that lies in between the initial take off and return to the base line. The phases also depend upon the synchronous firing of the muscle fibers in the motor unit. Normal motor unit potential may be biphasic or triphasic. More number of phases is termed as polyphasia and this indicates abnormality (Fig. 14.1).

When the patient performs maximal voluntary contraction of a particular muscle then all the motor unit in that muscle fires together and this is displayed on the screen as interference pattern (Fig. 14.2).

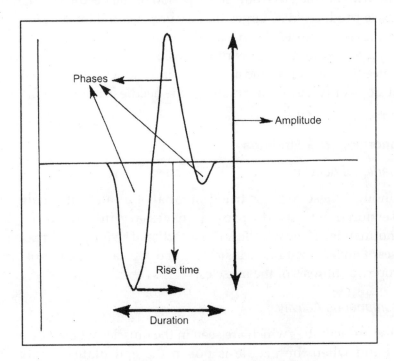

Fig. 14.1: Profile of a normal motor unit potential

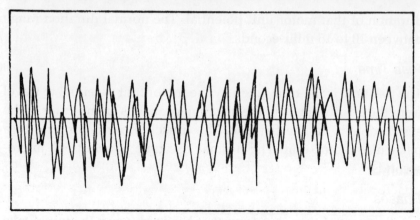

Fig. 14.2: Interference pattern

Interference pattern occurs because all the motor unit potentials get generated at the same time and appear in clusters making recognition of individual motor unit potential difficult. The potentials fill the whole screen to such an extent that the base line becomes invisible (Fig. 14.2).

Although a routine EMG recording is done only in the above mentioned methods its should be noted that when the recording is done with needle electrode, the invasion of the needle through the muscle produces discharges that occurs due to damage caused to the muscle by the piercing needle this is called as "*Insertional activity*". They are produced as a brief run of positive or negative spikes when the needle is in motion and also every time the needle is repositioned but stops or ceases off the moment the needle is held stationary or static.

Abnormal EMG Findings

Insertional Activity

Although these are not true potentials but an abnormality in insertional activity do provide necessary insight into some abnormalities of the muscles. The insertional activity is increased in cases of muscle membrane instability and decreased in cases of gross atrophy or fibrosis of the muscles.

Spontaneous Activity

These are activities which are seen in the muscles when they are at rest and when the needle is not in the end plate activity. To distinguish between abnormal spontaneous activity and normal end plate activity, one has to reposition the electrode to see whether these abnormal activities are reproduced. Spontaneous activities are seen between 2 and 4 weeks following a denervation when the muscle end plate becomes hypersensitive to acetylcholine by 100 folds. This phenomenon known as denervation hypersensitivity may explain spontaneous discharges of denervated muscle fibers in response to small quantities of circulating Ach. The disappearance of fibrillation potential in artificially induced ischemia and in isolated muscle fibers also supports the presence of some circulating substance. Spontaneous activity if reproduced at least two or 3 sites on the muscle provides an unequivocal sign of abnormality. Spontaneous activity when observed in patient with lower motor neuron presentation then its distribution may help in localizing lesion in the spinal cord, plexus or peripheral nerve. In certain acute upper motor neuron lesions, spontaneous activity may be seen in muscles between 6 weeks and 3 months. The spontaneous activity can take any one of the following forms:

Fibrillation potential: These are predominant negative potential with a very small initial positivity. The size of the fibrillation potential range from 20 to 200 microvolts in amplitude and 1 to 5 ms in duration when recorded with a concentric needle electrode. These resembles the end plate activity activity and hence one should known to discriminate. Repositioning of the needle helps in confirming the existence of end plate in the muscles. Fibrillation potential produces a characteristic sound on the loud speaker which is that of rain drop falling on tin roof or crisping sound of a crumbling aluminium foil. Although fibrillation potential has been associated with neurologic lesions, it may also be seen in certain muscular dystrophy due to secondary muscular denervation.

Positive sharp waves (Fig. 14.3): These are predominantly positive potential in which there is an initial positive phase of larger amplitude and shorter duration followed by negative spike of a longer duration and shorter amplitude giving the potential a saw tooth appearance. Therefore this potential is also called as *saw tooth potential*. They may be seen immediately following insertion of the needle but may also fire spontaneously. Like fibrillation potentials, positive sharp waves are also seen mainly in denervated muscles.

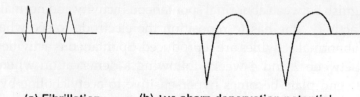

(a) Fibrillation   (b) +ve sharp denervation potential

Fig. 14.3: Positive sharp waves

However, certain myogenic conditions like polymyositis, dermato-myositis and progressive muscular dystrophy, may also show fibrillation potential.

Presence of fibrillation potentials and positive sharp waves can be quantified in clinical study into grades as follows:

+1 Transient but reproducible runs of positive discharge after moving the needle electrode which is also called as insertional positive waves.

+2 Occasional spontaneous potentials at rest in more than two different sites.

+3 Spontaneous activities present at rest in more than two different sites.

+4 Abundant spontaneous potentials nearly filling the screen of the oscilloscope.

Fasciculation potential or myokymic discharges:

Fasciculation potentials result from spontaneous discharges of a group of muscle fibers representing either a whole or possibly part of a motor unit. Motor unit potentials in the depth of the muscle may not necessarily induce visible twitches that can be seen by naked eyes. Under this circumstances electromyography becomes beneficial because of its ability to detect this invisible twitches and display on the screen as fasciculation potential. It may sometimes persist after distal nerve block. After total removal of the nerve supply to the muscle, fasciculation remains for about 4 days and then disappear. Then these fasciculation potentials appear like a normal motor unit potential but they occur spontaneously at a irregular rate and abnormal rhythm.

In contrast to fasciculation potential which involves isolated discharges of one motor unit, more complex bursts of repetitive discharges is called as myokymia. Repetitive firing of the same motor units usually occur in bursts at regular intervals of 0.1 to 10 seconds with 2 to 10 spikes discharging at 30 to 40 impulses per seconds in each burst.

Fasciculation potential although typically seen in anterior horn cell diseases are also seen in radiculopathy, entrapment neuropathy and muscular pain fasciculation syndrome. Fasciculation potential can also appear in some metabolic disorders like tetany, thyrotoxicosis, and over doses of anticholinesterase medications. Myokymic discharges on the other hand is seen in facial muscles in patients with brainstem glioma, or multiple sclerosis and in chronic neuropathies like Guillain Barré syndrome.

Complex repetitive discharge (Fig. 14.4): The repetitive discharge range from 50 microvolts to 1 millivolts in amplitude and up to 50 to 100 ms in duration. It represents synchronous firing of a group of muscle fibers. This discharge begins suddenly maintain a constant rate of firing for a short period and cease as abruptly as it started. Over the loud speaker this discharge produces a typical sound of a gun machine. They are some-what similar to the myotonic discharges but lack the typical waxing and waning. This discharge is seen in wide variety of chronic denervating conditions like motor neuron disease, radiculopathy, chronic polyneuropathy and Schwartz-Jampel syndrome.

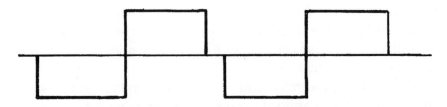

Fig. 14.4: Complex repetitive discharge

Abnormalities in the motor unit potentials: As discussed earlier in the chapter that certain parameter like amplitude, duration, phases are quite significant in describing the motor units potentials. Infact these parameters are very contributory in determining an abnormality of the motor unit profile and carries a great deal of clinical importance in differentiating between muscular pathology (myopathies) and nerve pathology (neuropathy). Although EMG may be inefficient in highlighting the type of nerve and muscular problem but when combined with certain other useful electrophysiological procedures like NCV, late response and evoked potential the outcome of the whole analysis will definitely lead the investigation towards a very conclusive brink from where the diagnosis is a lot easier. The motor unit abnormalities is quite contrast in neurogenic and in myogenic conditions mainly because of the way a certain change progress in these two vital organs. While nerve has a great deal of flexibility when it comes to compensation and irreversibility of the disorders, muscles on the other hand have a very poor compensatory abilities with irreversible changes. The abnormal findings in case of myopathies and neuropathies is as follows.

Neuropathies or Neurogenic Conditions

Lower motor neurons like polyneuropathies, motor neuron diseases, syringomyelia, polio and recovering peripheral nerve injury generally show motor unit potentials which are larger than normal in amplitude and longer in duration. Increase in amplitude occurs because most of the time in neuropathies when a particular axon or nerve cell is damaged the neighboring axon compensates by sending out collaterals to innervate those muscle fibers which was initially innervated by the damaged axon. This increases the motor unit density and motor unit territory which in turn causes an increase in the amplitude and duration. Apart from the motor unit territory, the difference in the length of the regenerating axon and extent of their myelination also contributes towards increasing the duration of the resultant potential.

The process is illustrated in the Figures 14.5A and B. Figures 14.5A and B indicates a simplified version of the arrangement of muscle fibers with their axon in a small cross sectional area of a muscle. The Figure 14.5A shows muscle fibers which are innervated by three different axons A, B,C thus constituting three different motor units. When A and C gets degenerated as shown in Figure 14.5B, "B" sends terminal collaterals to supply some of the muscle fibers which were initially supplied by A and B thus its size increases by two to three folds as shown in Figure 14.6 for interference in neuropathy. Consequently C which is quite giant motor unit also produces giant motor unit potential on EMG testing.

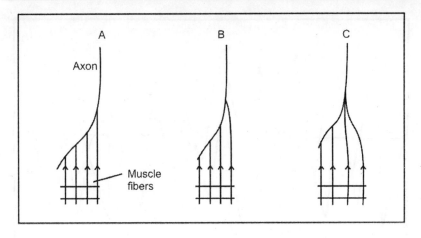

Fig. 14.5A: Showing three motor units constituted by 3 motor axons, A,B and C and its innervation to muscle fibers

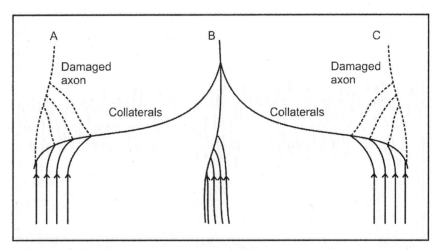

Fig. 14.5B: Showing as A and C are damaged or degenerated axon, "B" sends collaterals to the muscle fibers of A and C, thus increasing the size of its motor unit

Myopathies or Myogenic Conditions

In myopathies because the muscle fiber size and number reduces, the motor unit become small in size and weak. As the motor unit density and the motor unit territory both reduces the amplitude and duration of the displayed potential is less as compared to normal potential.

Phases are determined by the synchronous firing of the muscle fibers and its axons. As in both myopathy and neuropathy, there is

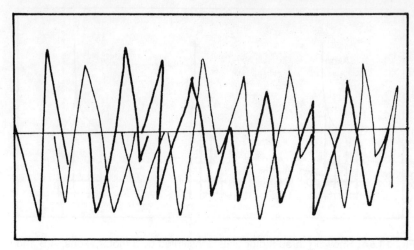

Fig. 14.6: Interference pattern in neuropathy (incomplete interference)

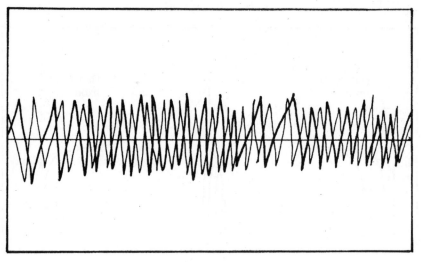

Fig. 14.7: Interference pattern in myogenic disorder (Early but complete)

asynchronous discharge it affects the phases of the motor unit potential giving rise to polyphasia.

Abnormality in the recruitment pattern : Under normal circumstances recruitment is proportional to the extent of contraction of the muscle. Maximum recruitment is a stage when all the motor unit in the muscle fires to their maximum possible limit in response to the maximal resistance applied to the muscle. In myopathy as the individual motor unit has reduced in size and strength they are recruited early to compensated for the lesser force exerted by an individual motor unit. Thus even for resistance which is much less than the maximal resistance all the motor units in the muscle fires to overcome the resistance giving rise to early but complete interference. The size of the motor unit will be small (Fig. 14.7).

NERVE CONDUCTION STUDIES

Dawson and Scott developed a reliable technique of determining mixed nerve conduction using better resolution, initially using photographic superimposition and later by electrical averaging. Dawson also recorded pure sensory nerve action potential on the nerve trunk by stimulating the digital nerve using ring electrode worn in the digits of the subject. With steady improvement of recording apparatus, nerve conduction studies have become a simple and reliable test of peripheral function

Nerve conduction studies is a diagnostic procedure which studies the conduction velocity of the peripheral nerve by electrically stimulating the nerve and finding the time taken by the impulses to travel from the point of stimulation to recording point or between two site of stimulation. Thus the measurement of conduction depends upon the proper analysis of the compound potential generated from the muscle in case of motor conduction velocity and from the nerve trunk in case of sensory conduction velocity.

Stimulators

Either a constant voltage or constant current stimulators can be used. The shape of the impulse should be square, and not triangular, to prevent accommodation of the nerve. The pulse duration range from 0.05 to 1.0 ms. Surface stimulation of 0.1 ms pulse duration with a intensity of 100 to 300 V or 5 to 40 mA is usually sufficient to activate a healthy nerve. Diseased nerve may need an intensity of upto 400 to 500 V or 60 to 75 mA. Although the above intensity range is quite safe under normal circumstances, however in patient with cardiac pacemaker, central venous pressure lines, indwelling cardiac catheters the procedures is usually avoided.

Electrodes

There are stimulating electrode, recording electrodes and ground electrodes for proper earthing.

Stimulating electrodes are bipolar (anode and cathode fixed to the single piece) non-invasive needle electrodes. As the current flows between the poles, cathode causes depolarization of the nerve with hyperpolarization under the anode. Thus in bipolar stimulation the cathode should be held distal to the anode on the nerve trunk to prevent the impulses from having anodal block. The alternative way is to place the anode off the nerve trunk to prevent blocking of the impulse generated.

The recording electrodes are always two surface electrode with one being the active and the other reference. Surface electrodes are better than needle electrodes for recording compound evoked potential. In case of motor conduction studies, accuracy of conduction velocity calculation depends a lot on the proper measurement of the distance between the consecutive cathodal points used to stimulate the nerve at multiple site. The distance between the two stimulation points should be strictly measured from cathode to cathode and not cathode to anode or vice versa.

Method for Motor Conduction Velocity

Electrode Placement

The stimulating electrode is placed on the nerve trunk with the cathode held closer to the recording site and distal to the anode. This arrangement is essential to prevent anodal blockade of the impulses.

The recording electrode is placed in such a way that the active electrode is placed on the muscle bulk and the reference is place either on the tendon of the recording muscle or on a nearby bony prominences.

The distance between the stimulating and recording electrode should not be too short while the distance between the active and reference electrode should not be too far in order to keep the stimulus artifact to the minimum.

The ground electrode is placed between the stimulating electrode and the recording electrode to diminish the stimulus artifact.

Patient Preparation

The part to be tested should be wiped with alcohol to dry skin that has some moisture as a result of perspiration. Adequate preparation of the stimulating and recording site reduces the skin resistance. Surface grease will dissolve if cleaned with ether. Callous skin needs gentle abrasion with dull knife or fine sandpaper. Rubbing the skin with a cream or solvent of high conductance lowers the impedance between the electrode and the underlying tissue.

Amplifier Settings

The gain set in the amplifier should be appropriate that it helps in accurate recording. Overamplification causes truncating of the peak of the evoked potential whereas inadequate amplification leads to inaccurate measurements.

Stimulating and Recording Procedures

For motor conduction velocity, the nerve is stimulated at two or three points. The stimulating electrode is held on the nerve in such a manner that the anode is 2 to 3 cm proximal to the cathode. Depolarization under the cathode results in generation of an impulse whereas hyperpolarization under the anode causes block to the propagation of the nerve impulse. This blocking of the impulse by anode is called as anodal block. The recording electrodes are placed in the manner mentioned above. When the stimulating current is increased in intensity it causes activation of the muscle innervated by the nerve which is stimulated. This activation is recorded by the active recording electrode that is placed on or near the motor point of the muscle bulk. The recorded muscle potential is a simple biphasic wave with a initial negativity. In case the recording electrodes are not properly positioned it may cause a very small positive peak preceding the negative peak. The displayed activity is freezed and then certain parameters like latency, amplitude and duration is measured.

Latency is measured from the stimulus artifact to the onset of the negative response. Amplitude is measured from the peak of the negative phase to the peak of the positive phase. Duration is measured from the initial take off of the wave to its return to the base line.

The latency measured in a motor conduction velocity studies consists of two components:
1. Nerve conduction time from the stimulus point to the nerve terminal.
2. Neuromuscular transmission, from the axon terminal across to the motor end plate including the time taken for generation of muscle action potential.

To measure the conduction velocity across the nerve trunk it is necessary to eliminate the time taken for neuromuscular transmission and for generation of the motor potential. Hence stimulation at two different site along the nerve trunk is necessary. The difference in the latency between proximal and distal stimulation nullifies the time taken at the neuromuscular junction as it happens to be a common pathway for proximal and distal stimulation. Thus the latency difference represents the time taken by the impulse to travel between the proximal and distal stimulation. The conduction velocity can now be derived using the formula Distance/ time, which is as follows:

$$\text{MCV} = \text{Distance} / \text{time} = \text{D in mm} / \text{Lp - Ld in ms} = \text{D} / \text{Lp - Ld m} / \text{s}$$

Here D is the distance between the proximal and distal point of stimulation, Lp and Ld are latency proximal and latency distal respectively (Fig. 14.8).

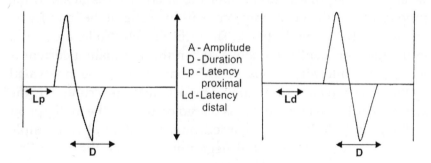

Fig. 14.8: MCV

Clinical Interpretation of MCV (Motor Conduction Velocity)

It has been noted that demyelination causes a decrease in the conduction velocity whereas axonal degeneration causes a decrease in the amplitude. Three basic types of abnormality pertaining to the latency and amplitude can be noted which are as follows:

- *Reduced amplitude with normal or slight increase in the latency:* When the nerve is simulated above the site of lesion and recorded below it produces a reduced amplitude but when stimulated below, the site of lesion it produces a normal motor potential. If this is seen in the first few days following a nerve lesion it is not possible to differentiate between neurapraxia and axonotmesis. However after few days in axonotmesis the part of the nerve below the site of lesion also starts getting degenerated causing a reduction in amplitude. Infact this deterioration in the amplitude will keep progressing till the degeneration process in complete. Once regeneration starts the muscle which is innervated early will start showing an improvement in its potential. Thus regular assessment is essential in nerve conduction velocity studies.

Partial neurapraxia is indicated if the amplitude of the potential obtained after distal stimulation is less than the amplitude of the potential obtained after proximal stimulation without any further deterioration in the amplitude as in axonotmesis. Moreover stimulation above and below the site of lesion will cause potential with equal amplitude in axonotmesis. Thus it is possible to discriminate a neurapraxic lesion from an axonotmesis although the abnormality may appear similar.

- *Increase in the conduction time (decrease in the conduction velocity) with a normal amplitude of the motor potential:* These changes generally suggestive of segmental neuropathy. A prolonged latency or decreased conduction velocity may also result from axonal neuropathy of the fast conducting nerve fibers in the peripheral nerve. Involvement of the axon will also cause a reduction in the amplitude of the motor potential along with decrease in the conduction velocity. Motor conduction velocity may also reduce in cases of anterior horn cell loss as seen in myelopathies.

    Assuming that there are no technical errors, if proximal and distal stimulation produces dissimilar wave form from the same nerve then their latencies may represents two groups of motor fibers with different conduction characteristics in the same nerve.

- *Absent response:* When the nerve is stimulated proximal to the site of involvement and recording is done distally fails to produce a response then it can indicate a complete neurapraxia or complete neurotmesis. Distal stimulation will produce a normal response in both conditions for the first one weeks, but later on there will be deterioration in neurotmesis which may not be seen in neurapraxia. The difference between the two conditions becomes evident because neurapraxia will show signs of improvement whereas complete neurotmesis will not produce any response.

Sensory Conduction Velocity Testing

For sensory conduction velocity, one can use either antidromic impulse or orthodromic impulse for studying their conduction. For sensory nerves, the antidromic impulse travel towards the distal direction whereas orthodromic travel towards the spinal cord. However studying the orthodromic flow of impulse is considered more often.

The stimulating electrodes are ring electrodes that is worn in the appropriate digit and recording is done directly from the nerve trunk. The recording electrode is a surface electrode that will record the sensory potential directly from the nerve. The recording electrodes are two active which is placed directly on the nerve trunk and reference that is placed at a remote area.

The intensity of the stimulus is increased gradually till the sensory nerve action potential reaches to its maximum amplitude such that any further increase in the intensity of the stimulus fails to cause a increase in the amplitude of the potential. The sensory potential appear as triphasic wave form with initial positivity. Placing the reference electrode near the nerve at a distance of more than 3 cm will make the recorded potential tetraphasic with a final negativity.

The amplitude, latency, duration and wave form of the potential is studied. The conduction velocity can be calculated as follows (Fig. 14.9):

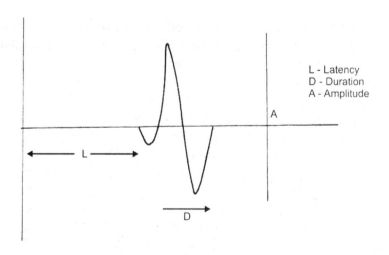

L - Latency
D - Duration
A - Amplitude

Fig. 14.9: SCV

SCV = Distance / Time = D/ Latency in mm/ms = m/s

The abnormalities applicable for motor conduction velocity can also be applied for sensory conduction studies.

Factor Affecting Conduction Velocity of a Nerve

- Increased temperature increases the speed of conduction whereas-cooling reduces it.
- Nerves in the lower limb conduct slowly as compared to nerves in the upper limb.
  Longer nerves generally conducts very slowly as compared to shorter nerves. The nerve impulse also propagates faster in cases of proximal segment of the nerve in comparison to the distal segments.
- The nerve propagation doubles from infancy to about 5 years due to the rapid myelination that is seen in all the nerves of the body. In later childhood and adolescence, the conduction velocity in the upper limb increases whereas that in the lower limb shows a decrease. After about 40 years there is a gradual decline in the conduction velocity of all the nerves in the body.
- Other factors like ischemia, also causes a slowing of the nerve conduction velocity.

F Wave

F wave is a late response that results due to back firing of antidromic impulse when a supramaximal stimulus is applied on the peripheral nerve. This late response occur after the direct muscle response and was first observed by Magladery and Macdougal.

Production of F Wave

When a supramaximal stimulus is applied over the nerve, impulses are produced in two direction, an orthodromic impulse which travel directly to the muscle to produce the M response and the antidromic impulse which travel in antidromic direction towards the spinal cord. This antidromic impulse doesn't travel through the usual reflex pathway but turn backward from the anterior horn cell via the same motor axon to produce potential in the innervated muscle which is termed as F wave. The presence of F wave in differentiated limbs proves that the transportation of impulse takes place only in the motor axon without any contribution from the sensory axon.

Recurrent discharge of F wave with repeated stimulation of the same nerve may not always produce as in some motor units the impulse fails to end the somata as they get blocked by the axon hillock.

Latency

With distal stimulation, the F wave is always produced after the M response. The time taken to produce the F wave is called F latency and the time taken to produce M response is called as M latency. Thus usually the F latency is more than the M latency. As the point of stimulation moves more and more proximal the latency of F wave becomes lesser and lesser whereas that of M response becomes more and more. Infact, at the axilla the F wave and the M wave overlap. In such cases simultaneous stimulation is given at the wrist and the axilla so that the antidromic impulses at the wrist and the orthodromic impulses from the axilla collide thus allowing production of M response at the wrist and F wave at the axilla. F latency at the axilla can also be calculated as

$$F \text{ (axilla)} = F \text{ (wrist)} + M \text{ (wrist)} - M \text{ (axilla)}$$

There exist latency difference between the successive F wave produced in the same nerve with repeated stimulation of the same intensity which is in the range of 10 to 30 microseconds. This difference in the latency is because of the difference in the conduction time across the faster conducting and slower conduction axon. Conduction time is not only the measure of the speed at which the impulses travel but also the length of the axon. The axon terminal differ in their length depending upon the position of the motor end plate and this could be an important contributing factor which varies the length of the axon. Moreover the tip of the axon terminal is unmyelinated which further contributes to slowing the conduction of the impulse across them. The position of the recording electrode with respect to the motor unit also determines the latency of the F wave.

Although the amplitude and duration are not as clinically significant as the latency but they do give information regarding the motor neuron excitability.

Recording of F Wave

Machine settings

- Gain: 100 to 500 microvolts per cm
- Sweep: 5 to 10 milliseconds per cm
- Amplitude: Supramaximal
- Electrode position: Stimulating electrode consists of anode and cathode. The cathode is place at the stimulating site on the nerve trunk whereas anode is kept off the nerve trunk to prevent anodal block. The recording electrode consists of active and reference electrodes. The active electrode is placed on the muscle bulk whereas the reference is placed on the tendon of the same muscles.

With each stimuli F wave is produced after the direct M response. The earliest and late latency of the successive F wave is a measure of temporal dispersion. Electronic averaging helps in finding the mean F latency of a specific nerve.

With distal stimulation F latency gives information regarding conduction time along entire motor axon. Thus F latency becomes very informative in diffuse and multisegmental lesion where routine nerve conduction velocity studies fail to show significant reduction in the conduction ability of the nerve (Fig. 14.10).

For all practical purposes the ulnar and median nerve are studied by stimulating at the wrist and elbow in the upper limb whereas the common peroneal and the tibial are studied by stimulating at the ankle and knee in the lower limb.

Factors Influencing F Wave

- Mild voluntary contraction during stimulation of the recording muscles enhances production of F wave but maximum voluntary contraction causes collision between the volitional impulses and the antidromic impulses thus preventing the generation of F wave.
- Dentate nucleus stimulation abolishes F wave.
- Intramuscular and intravenous injection facilitate production of F wave.
- Increase in thyrotropic releasing hormone also facilitate F wave.

Clinical Implication of F wave

- In case of Guillain Barré syndrome the proximal portion of the nerve may show increase in the F latency.

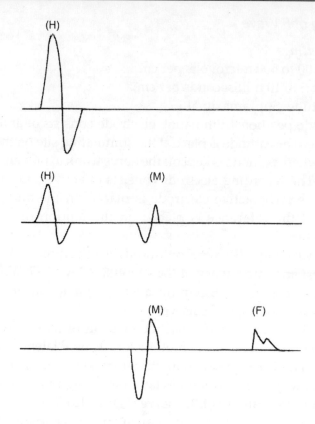

Fig. 14.10: Change in response as the stimules progresses from threshold to supramaximal

- In mild cases of hereditary sensory motor neuropathy the distal portion of the nerve may show increase in the F latency but in advance cases the entire portion of the nerve may show increase in the F latency.
- Radiculopathy or plexopathy involving the motor roots will show increase in the F latency when the routine nerve conduction velocity studies along the peripheral portion of the involved nerve will show normal results.
- The ulnar and median nerve may show involvement in syringomyelia.
- Even in diabetic and uremic neuropathy the F latency may be involved.
- The F ratio which is F latency divided by M latency show a fall due to involvement of median nerve in Carpal tunnel syndrome.

H Reflex

Reflex studies gives information regarding the conduction along the afferent pathway, efferent pathway as well as spinal motor neuron excitability. Neurological examination that tests the reflex clinically like deep tendon jerks gives information about the motor neuron excitability along with finding out the continuity of the reflex arc but the limitation of these clinical examination lies in the fact that they don't quantify the response obtained and hence at times becomes subjective. Electrically studied spinal monosynaptic reflex activity called as H reflex or Hoffmann's reflex. It involves stimulating a peripheral nerve with maximal stimulus such that the impulses travel through the normal spinal monosynaptic reflex pathway to produce contraction of the innervated muscles.

In newborn babies and infants upto first year of life it is possible to elicit H reflex in all the peripheral nerves. But in adults one can practically elicit H reflex only in the calf muscles and in the flexor carpi radialis. As the intensity of stimulation progresses from sub-threshold to supramaximal the H reflex reaches its peak during maximal stimulation after which the intensity of H reflex gradually reduces until and unless it is eventually replaced by the M response and F wave. The M response and F wave are produced due to orthodromic and antidromic impulse produced in the motor axon as the intensity progresses from maximal to supramaximal causing direct stimulation of the motor axon. The reason for the H reflex to get extinct with higher intensity of stimulation can be theoretically given as follows:

- Collision between the antidromic impulse and H reflex impulse in the alpha motor neuron
- Refractory period of the axon hillock following entry of antidromic impulse into the cell body which prevents the H reflex impulse from traveling down the alpha motor neuron
- Probable Renshaw cell inhibition via intermediate neurons to the same motor neuron and even the neighboring axon.

Unlike F wave, which showed different latency and wave form with successive stimulation, the H reflex doesn't change with repeated stimulation as the same motor neurons produces the impulses.

It reflex can be obtained from tibial nerve as follows:

Recording procedure

The patient may be asked to lie prone but the preferable position is making the patient sit in such a manner that the knee is flexed to about 120 degree with the foot relaxed and resting on the floor. A force plate may be kept under the sole to record the force exerted by the foot. A potentiometer may be attached to the ankle to study the degree of movement at the ankle joint.

Recording electrode

The recording electrode may be kept at any of the two site based upon the necessity. If the response is to be recorded from the entire calf muscles then the active electrode is placed over the tendo Achilles 2 cm distal to the point of insertion of the tendon Achilles whereas the reference electrode is placed 3 cm distal to the active electrode.

In case the recording is to be done from the soleus muscle then the active electrode is placed half way between the tibial tuberosity and the medial malleolus whereas the reference is placed over the tendon medial and proximal to the medial malleolus.

The ground electrode is placed in between the stimulating electrode and the recording electrode. The activity of the antagonist which in this case is the tibialis anterior can be recorded by placing a recording electrode over the tibialis anterior.

Stimulation can be any of the following ways:

- Electrical stimulation using a bipolar electrode placed on the tibial nerve in the popliteal fossa. This being the most common type of stimulation produced
- Sudden stretch applied to the tendon Achilles.
- Mechanical tap produced by a neurological hammer that is attached to the oscilloscope.

The H reflex obtained following such stimulation can be biphasic with initial negativity if recorded from soleus or triphasic with initial positivity when recorded from the tendon Achilles.

Clinical Implication

- H reflex testing is used to obtain a quantified data of the degree of spasticity for various research activity.
- It records conduction along the entire reflex pathway and hence important in assessment of upper motor and lower motor neuron lesion.

It is depressed or absent in various diabetic neuropathy and even radiculopathy.

SELF-ASSESSING QUESTIONS

- Explain the parameter of normal EMG.
- Explain abnormal EMG.
- Describe EMG findings in neurogenic and myogenic conditions.
- Explain the method of doing motor and sensory conduction velocity studies.
- Write a note on F latency.
- Write a short note on H reflex.
- Write a note on spontaneous activity.
- Write a note on interference pattern.

15

Common Approaches in Neurorehabilitation

As a therapist, one comes across various types of neurological disorders with various types of presentation that in turn causes different types of functional limitations. However, if one carefully notices the common problems that contribute maximally to functional limitation and needs a greater physiotherapy role then it has to be weakness, abnormal tonicity and improper control. Thus most of the patients limitation due to neurological disorders is centered around these abnormalities. Hence most of the approaches is targeted either to increase the strength or improve the control or normalize the tone.

Before knowing what techniques that needs to be used, one should know the principles on the basis of which the treatment techniques produce results. The beauty of the various physiotherapy approaches in neurological disorder is its ability to bring about the necessary adaptation required in the central nervous system or even in the peripheral nervous system which contributes towards the achievements. Of course our brain has the ability of mould itself at any age depending upon the various stimulus given or the demand put in due to the ability that is called a *Neuroplasticity* but this natural process can be facilitated to a greater extent by physiotherapy interventions.

Plasticity is a general term used to describe the tendency to modify or be flexible so as to get adapted to a changed environment. Thus neuroplasticity is the ability of the brain and neural structures to adapt themselves after its disruption so as to reorganize themselves which in turn helps in regaining their function to variable extent.

During neural plasticity there is a continuum from short term changes in the efficiency or strength of synaptic connections to long term structural changes in the organization and numbers of connections among neurons.

We know that the development process which takes place from our birth leads to formation of neurological circuits which is essential to carry out the learned function. Each an every activity we learn during our growth (eating, dressing, walking, combing, etc.) leads to formation of a neurological organization representing a particular activity which makes these activities automatic so that one doesn't have to necessarily concentrate on it. This neurological organization is termed as *Engram*. Engram is defined as a neurological organization of preprogrammed pattern such that every time an engram for a specific task is activated the task is carried out automatically. Due to neuronal damage this engram is disrupted causing inability to perform previously learned task. However due to the tendency of neuronal plasticity, the brain has the ability to once again relearn the lost activity by forming new engram by making use of redundant cells and neuron but the extent of this ability may vary depending upon various factors. The recovery seen in stroke is a classical example of the brain's ability to learn the lost activity.

During a normal living one does not use all the available neurons in the central nervous system. This is because some of the cells and neurons in our brain and spinal cord are called as redundant neurons which have a higher level of excitation and hence they don't get stimulated during the normal developmental process because of which they don't contribute for the various activities performed by a person. Various physiotherapy interventions reach the threshold level of excitations of the redundant neurons so that they take on the function of the damaged neurons. The extent and the rate at which this prognosis takes place depends upon the various factors like extent of lesion, age of the patient, motivation of the patient, type and skill of the physiotherapy interventions.

For the lower motor neuron types of disorder the real challenge to the therapist is to maintain the muscle properties and keep the atrophy to the minimum. Because the changes in the muscles is irreversible hence if the muscle fibers reduces in number then even with restoration of neuronal connection the muscle will not be able to generate the maximum power which it generates under normal circumstances.

VARIOUS APPROACHES

It is essential one is quite familiar with the various types of approaches used for neurological disorders and they are as follows:
1. Neurodevelopmental approaches
2. Sensory integration
3. PNF
4. Motor relearning program
5. Biofeedback
6. Strengthening techniques
7. Barnstorm techniques
8. Margaret Rood's technique

Neurodevelopmental Approaches

This approach of neurorehabilitation that originated way back in 1940 was developed by Dr Karl Bobath and his wife Berta Bobath PT, physiotherapist. This approach evolved as a response to the need for more effective treatment of children with cerebral palsy. This treatment technique wads discovered from clinical experiences of these therapists and developed over time to deal with the treatment of patients with abnormal movements. Berta found that handling the patient's body made a difference in the distribution of stiffness and control of movement. This became the inception of neuro facilitation techniques used in treatment today.

Through Berta's clinical experience her husband began to explain the phenomena of responses and recovery her patients exhibited and thus the *Neuro-developmental Therapy Approach* began to emerge.

One of the important contributions from this area of practice was the description of normal and abnormal movement as a basis for analyzing motor control.

The theoretical explanation of this approach used the current neurological research of its day. Reflex hierarchy theory was in vogue and became the basis for defining and explaining neurological symptoms. The problems in cerebral palsy were felt to be the result of a release of abnormal postural reflexes and tone which interfered with the development of higher-level reactions and equilibrium responses. Righting and equilibrium reactions became the hallmarks of the highest level of skill attainable using this approach. A hierarchical approach to recovery and development was adopted.

Sensory information was also regarded in this theory as playing an important part in the development of motor control. Abnormal experience was felt to provide abnormal feedback and interfered with the development of learning more functional ability.

As this technique was getting developed it was found that there was a need to do a preliminary analysis of movement before implementing the treatment process. Analysis of the patient's movement was based on observation and was compared to normal developmental sequences. Contrasting abnormal movement with normal was described. Abnormal movement patterns were described as primitive reflex responses which has lost its higher influences. These responses were categorized and labeled. Clinical approaches developed using techniques to inhibit reflex responses and facilitate more normal activity, such as those seen in higher-level responses and reactions, i.e. righting and equilibrium. A process of inhibiting abnormal responses was integrated with facilitation techniques to produce more normal control.

Off late the development of new motor learning and motor control theories it is shown that the nervous system no longer functions as a set of rules but has multiple parallel and distributed influences in the development of postural control. These fields of theoretical basis have begun to rule out the earlier belief that motor system functions as a independent unit but have proved with experiments that it depends upon many systems. Thus motor learning and expressions needs the contribution from various areas to function effectively. Sensory information continues to be considered a valid influence on movement. This body of research has modified the explanation of how a patient controls movement and relearns control. NDT theory has broadened some of the approaches used in the treatment of neurological recovery because of new findings. The Neurodevelopmental Treatment Association has adopted current information into their approach as explanation for intervention and recovery. Reflexes are no longer the focus of the fight. Analysis of movement continues as the central part of the evaluation format. The use of handling techniques remains the tool used to inhibit undesirable and inefficient postural control. Facilitation of more functional control of movement remains the goal of this approach. The context of the functional task and the environmental demands are now more emphasized in therapy than was previously described.

To date there has been no formal standardized testing developed by the NDT Association. There are some qualitative movements based exams that have been developed in recent years and are now emerging on the market. Norm referenced and standardized tests of gross and fine motor performance continue to provide a guide to the therapist for functional performance. These tests are combined with this approach as a basis for examination with the inclusion of clinical observation of the quality of movement.

Sensory Integration

It has been proved on more than one occasion that sensory system has facilitatory or inhibitory influences on the motor system. Motor system doesn't function independently but needs input from various sensory systems. Over a period of time researcher have used various mode of sensory system like cutaneous sensation, proprioceptors, visual etc. to get the desired motor response. Sensory integration is the term used to indicate a therapeutic procedure, which combines various forms of sensory input to get the desired motor response. Sensory integration uses principles such as the following:

- *Vestibular based activities:* It is given by means of a movable surfaces like vestibular ball or tilt board which helps to stimulate the patient's righting reactions, equilibrium reaction and automatic adaptation responses. Thus this exercises helps in improving the balance, postural control, weight shifts, muscle tone and coactivation of different groups of muscles. These activities also improves the protective extension activity thus promoting self control and security with movements.
- *Tactile based activities:* It helps to facilitate body scheme and body image awareness. The various modes of tactile inputs that can be given is deep and light pressure input, use of brushing, application of lotions, pressure garments and self-controlled tactile experiences. Tactile stimulation helps in improving the discriminatory responses and decreases defensiveness.
- *Proprioceptive:* Various activities that stimulate the proprioceptors are weight bearing activities, stretching, high impact activities like climbing and jumping. Proprioceptive stimulation facilitates organization of neuromuscular system, coactivation of muscle groups, integration and regulation of modulatory responses and body perception which are necessary component of feedback for motor learning.

- *Coordination activities:* It uses activities which incorporates timing of responses, pairing of vision with motor outcomes and ability to localize or target an area for accuracy as well as grading of muscular activation patterns. This activity helps to facilitate control of rate rhythm and timing of muscular activation. The various activities which are used are finger tapping, skipping, jumping, hopping, kicking ball, catching ball, hitting a ball, writing are some of the examples.
- *Visual motor:* Ocular motor skills, localization, tracking, scanning, gaze shift, visual spatial analysis, transitional adjustments in postural control are obtained with these activities. The activity selected should combine active ocular control with vestibular-based activities in order to integrate ocular motor skill and eye-hand activities. Visual motor skills are essential for feed forward control, for developing anticipatory responses as well as for developing optical and head righting reactions.
- *Oral motor:* It uses activities which incorporates active motor control like blowing, bubbles, chewing, biting, various facial expression so that it facilitates range of motion of lips, tongue and jaw. This skill helps in facilitating swallowing, blowing, sucking, chewing and oral imitating in praxis.
- *Auditory:* It facilitates the perception of auditory information in a way to improve orienting responses as well as assist the motor system to learn how to use rhythm and timing during movement. Use of sound sources to create an outside rhythm to aid in the perception of timing in the control of movement. Music may regulate emotional modulation through the use of relaxation enticed through the use of sound. Rhythmic sounds helps in relaxing thus can be used to inhibit tone. Arrhythmic sounds on the other hand are alerting and hence can be used to have facilitatory effect on the tone of the muscles.
- *Olfactory:* It facilitates the integration of smell with gustatory responses and may create an alerting or calming responses in the patient.

Sensory integrative therapy can be best practised if it is carried out in a separate room where other external disturbance does not exist. Moreover rehabilitation of autistic child can be best achieved when the therapy is carried out in an isolated quiet room. The area should be large enough to provide opportunity for free movement sequences and allow the child self-exploration skill within his or her safety limits. The arrangement in the room should be consistently changed to prevent adaptation of the child which may remove the stimulating factors causing boredom. The equipment used in the room should provide sensory input and experiences, which will prove to be integral for motor and sensory processing. Certain equipments like swing, hammock, bolster, etc. can be suspended to stimulate the vestibular and proprioceptive apparatus. The equipment should be able to facilitate the motor planning ability of the child and should produce large muscle responses. The child should be given full freedom for executing motor tasks and activities like crawling, climbing, running and jumping should be encouraged. Other sensory inputs like tactile, auditory and visual should be incorporated into the activities of the child to improve attention, arousal, coordination, posture and balance.

The common equipments used in sensory integrative therapy consists of weights, swings, foams, bean bags, vibrators, turkey towel, cotton, brush, blankets, stairs, writing instruments, trapeze bars, platform, climbing toys, tunnels, large blocks, candies, balls, bolster, ramps, clays, etc.

Proprioceptive Neuromuscular Facilitation (PNF)

This technique to maneuver the motor response was introduced by Herman Kabat which was later on developed by Knott and Voss. It deals with making use of the proprioceptor to modify the action of the motor system. The main proprioceptor utilized for this purpose is the muscle spindle. The various principles which are used are:

- Stretch to stimulate the muscle spindle so as to facilitate contraction in the muscles
- Lumbrical grip is used to provide exteroception, stretch, resistance and traction or approximation
- The movement should be done in pattern because normal activities mostly occur in functional pattern due to the combined action of various muscles
- Over flow of impulses is possible for stronger muscles to weaker muscles or from stronger pattern to weaker pattern
- The patient should be made to work against maximal resistance to have beneficial effect

- Any movement combination causing functional pattern in the extremities is always initiated by the rotatory components followed by the distal most and then by the proximal part
- To stimulate the proprioceptors of the joint traction is given when the movement is done against gravity and approximation is given when the movement is done towards gravity
- Visual and verbal inputs are necessary hence the therapist should continuously give proper command and also should instruct the patient to look at the movement.

In rehabilitation of neurological conditions, PNF can be used for strengthening and lengthening. The strengthening techniques are Repeated contraction and Slow reversal.

Repeated contraction is further divided into normal timing, timing for emphasize and combination of isometric and isotonic work. Of these normal timing and timing for emphasize is used for neurological rehabilitation. In normal timing the therapist select a pattern which is weak and thus comes in the way of the functional independency hence this pattern needs to be strengthened. The selected pattern is repeated over and over again from the starting position to the end position. This technique is very effective when there is uniform or generalized weakness of a single pattern.

Timing for emphasize is used when there is patchy weakness of a specific muscle or group in a particular pattern. Thus there is weakness of a single component of the functional pattern that needs to be strengthened. Usually the joint across which the weak muscle lies is used as pivot and it is at this joint that the movement is encouraged. The movements at the joint distal and proximal to the pivot joint is restricted so that there is overflow of the impulses to the weaker muscle working at the pivot.

For lengthening or relaxation of spastic or shortened muscles, hold relax or contract relax is used. Here the spastic muscle is made to contract isotonically in contract relax technique and isometrically in hold relax technique so that strong contraction is followed by relaxation that in turn help in reducing spasticity or hypertonicity.

For rigidity, one can use rhythmic initiation technique in which the movement progresses from passive to active assisted to active so that the patient learns to initiate movement which out putting too much effort so that the tone of the muscle is kept in check.

For cases of hypotonicity in cerebellar disease, technique of rhythmic stabilization which involves alternately giving resistance to agonist and antagonist coupled with approximation so that it stimulate cocontraction of both the group of muscle which helps in improving fixation at a joint.

Motor Relearning Program (MRP)

This technique of developing motor control was introduced by Carr and Shepherd. According to this concept development of a functional task can be achieved best when the task itself is practiced on the whole in the original environment rather than developing other neurological factors like tone, strength or coordination in a position or setting that is totally different from the actual task. MRP is very effective in stroke patient and can be started as soon as the general medical condition of the patient stabilizes. Infact, motor rehearing program by itself is sufficient many a times in regaining control over various motor tasks. However other methods which involves either facilitating activity in a flaccid muscle or deactivating a hyperactive muscles (like Biofeedback) may be used in association with MRP in certain cases. Motor Relearning Program is practiced in four steps which are:

- Step 1 which involves thorough observation of the patient's performance of a functional task. Every functional task has various components that is necessary towards accomplishment of that task. Thus when the therapist observes the performance of the patient, he is in a position to list out those components that is missing in the patient's performance and is thus contributing towards the abnormal way of function. Then he needs to analyze the reason for the missing component. Detailed analysis can give sufficient information to the patient regarding associated problems, which can be anatomical, biomechanical, physiological and behavioral factors. Along with the other neurological assessment this observation and analysis gives direct information about the reason for dysfunction in a specific task. Checking tone, strength, control in supine may not produce enough information about these neurological parameters in the position and the body alignment in which a task is originally performed. Thus analysis of the reason for lack of various component in a particular functional task executed by the patient is very essential.

- Step 2 involves practice of the missing component using various visuals, verbal and manual feedback under the guidance of the therapist.
- Step 3 involves practice of the whole task using the same feedback as above.
- Step 4 consists of transfer of training during which the patient should maintain consistency in practice. The patient needs to practice the learned task in the environment of his home and when he is alone. The active participation of the family members and relatives during this period of motor relearning is very important. Lack of practice by the patient when he is alone may curtail the beneficial effect of the therapy.

Step 2 and 3 usually overlap, infact step 2 only comes into picture when the patient does not have a specific component like activity of certain muscle in which case, activation of this muscle is developed before the patient practices the whole activity.

A specific task is practiced as a whole. Only when a specific component of the task is missing should the patient be asked to practice the missing component. Infact once this missing component is activated immediately the patient should practice the whole activity. Tips given by the therapist will go a long way in helping the patient to understand the flaw in his performance, which in turn will help in rectification of the movement. Proper explanation and demonstration will help the patient in understanding as to why he is having difficulty in performing a task. Sometimes the therapist may have to use his manual guidance to move a limb into a specific position so that the patient does not have to struggle. For example, if the therapist is teaching the patient reaching upwards in supine position then she takes the arm into flexed position and is holding it to prevent it from internally rotating so that the patient is reminded to keep her elbow straight. The therapist can also use her manual guidance to provide spatial and temporal constraint. For example, the therapist may hold part of the limb to constrain the action spatially to allow the patient to generate a component on his own. Like for instance to make a patient assume standing from sitting, the therapist assist the patient in the first part of the movement by keeping his affected knee forward and pushing it posteriorly so that it will help the patient to anchor his foot to the ground and use his quadriceps and other extensors to assume standings the patient develops some control the therapist decreases her physical constraint so that the degrees of freedom which the patient has to control now increases. At this point in the training the manual assistance by the therapist should decreasing and verbal guidance is given instead.

Progression is very important, the patient should not keep practicing what he already can do. Activities should be progressed by making a specific task more complex by either decrease the guidance or by altering the speed, or by adding variety. Exposing the patient to different environmental conditions for a specific skill will help him to improve his performances. Last and the most important key is practice by the patient the new skill throughout the day.

Biofeedback

The biofeedback used in rehabilitation of neurological patient is EMG biofeedback. It is done with the help of surface EMG electrodes which is placed on the muscle or muscle groups that needs to be activated or inhibited. The machine detects the electrical activity of the muscles in the form of integrated potentials, which is displaced on the screen in association with some auditory feedback. Unlike clinical EMG in biofeedback one displays the integrated response from many motor units of the same muscles. With the introduction of computerized machines, the displayed wave represents the average response of all the motor units from which the surface electrode has recorded.

The biofeedback machine can be used to strengthen weak muscles as well as relax a hypertonic muscle. For strengthening process the patient is instructed to concentrate on increasing the size of the displayed wave whereas for relaxing a spastic muscle the patient is instructed to try and reduce the size of the displayed wave. EMG biofeedback can be used very successfully in rehabilitating cases of lower motor neuron lesions like neuropathy, peripheral nerve injury, etc. as well as upper motor neuron lesions like stroke. With the introduction of cordless electrode it has become very easy to provide the patient the essential feedback during functional retraining of activities like eating, brushing, reaching out, walking, etc.

Strengthening Techniques

Strengthening muscles is quite important in lower motor neuron as well as upper motor neuron conditions. In lower motor neuron one has to strengthen the agonist muscles whereas in upper motor neuron one has to strengthen the muscle groups, which is antagonist to the spastic muscle. Strengthening is essential to bring about good balance between the agonist and antagonist. Strengthening can be achieved in various ways like weight bearing, resisted exercises using weight, springs, hydrotherapy, suspension therapy and by using manual resistance. Vigorous resisted exercises are however contraindicated in certain conditions like dystrophy, spinal muscular atrophy as these exercises can increase the damage to the muscles. One needs to follow the various principles like overload, specificity, progression, duration, frequency, complacency, motivation while designing a strengthening program.

Brunstorm Technique

The technique developed by Brunstorm produce motion by provoking primitive movement patterns of synergistic movement pattern which are observed in fetal life and after pyramidal lesion. This technique is quite extensively used to develop tone in flaccid stage of hemiplegia and in pure pyramidal lesion. The main features consists of:

- Reflex responses are used initially and later voluntary control of these reflex patterns is trained.
- Control of head and trunk is trained with stimulation of tonic neck reflexes like ATNRL, STNR, Tonic Lumbar and Tonic Labyrinthine reflexes. This is followed by stimulation of righting reflexes and later balance training.
- Associated reactions are used as a mean of developing activities (hyperextension of thumb produces relaxation of the finger flexors).

Margaret Rood's Technique

This technique which is used for facilitating and relaxing is based on the following principles:
- Afferent or sensory stimuli is used to influence motor responses
- The nerve and sensory receptors are classified according to the types, location, effect, response and distribution. Technique of stimulation such as stroking, brushing, ice, heating, pressure, bone pounding, slow and quick stretch, joint traction and approximation, are used to facilitate or inhibit the motor response.

- Muscles are classified according to their action as light working muscles (hand and finger muscles) or heavy working muscles (trunk muscles) and hence depending upon their classification appropriate stimuli for their actions are used.
- Various reflexes like TNR, TLR, vestibular reflexes and withdrawal patterns are used in the therapy.
- Ontogenetic developmental sequence is strictly followed in the application of stimuli. Hence the therapy is given in the order of total flexion or withdrawal pattern, rolling, pivot prone, on elbows, crawl, standing upright, and walking.
- Vital functions: Developmental sequence of respiration, sucking, swallowing, phonation, chewing and speech is followed.

The above given approaches are some of the common approaches which are used by the author to rehabilitate patients with various types of neurological disorders. However while treating a neurological cases one cannot have a fixed protocol as no two patients with same conditions exhibit similar manifestation. The treatment needs to be tailor-made for individual patients. The theoretical background should be associated with good innovative practical ideas to make the treatment session more interesting as well as more effective for the patient.

SELF-ASSESSING QUESTIONS

- What is neuroplasticity?
- What is principle of redundancy?
- Explain the principle underlying physiotherapy intervention in various neurological disorders.
- Explain NDT or neurodevelopment technique.
- Explain motor relearning.
- Explain sensory integration.
- What is the principle underlying Brunstorm technique?
- What is the rationale or principle underlying Rood's technique?
- Explain biofeedback.
- Explain principles and technique of PNF.

16

Fatigue Assessment

Fatigue or tiredness is defined as a state during which a person is unable to carry out a particular activity any longer after performing it repeatedly for some time.

FATIGUE

It is usually of two types: *Local* in which fatigue is noticed in isolated muscle (work out of a single muscles on dumb bells in gym) or *General* in which the fatigue is not localized to one or two muscles but to most of the muscle in the body, e.g. Marathon running, swimming or playing foot ball.

Local Fatigue

The fatigue of local muscles can be demonstrated by simple examples like if a specific muscle is made to contract voluntarily or artificially by current. It is noted that the initial few repetition of contraction helps in improving the performance of the muscle. In the sense it contracts much better because these initial few contraction act as a warm up which helps in:

- Acceleration of chemical reaction time
- Increases the catalytic ability of the enzymes
- Lowers the viscosity.

Moreover, various neurological factors like more synchronous recruitment and firing of the motor units helps in increasing the force of contraction with a less latency period.

Repeated contraction might also cause an increased calcium concentration within the fiber due to the phenomenon of summation and may further increase the contractility.

However these beneficial effects occurs only for the initial few repetitions and later on they are over. Infact if these contractions are continued then the muscle begins to show signs of fatigue. This can be explained considering three criterias which are as follows:

- Progressive increase of the latent period
- Progressive diminution of the height of contraction
- Increase in the phase of relaxation.

Later on a stage is reached when the muscles fails to produce a flicker or a twitch although the stimulation continues. Also since the muscle fails to relax completely there is chances of development of contracture.

The local fatigue that sets in is due to the changes in the muscles themselves. Merton (1954) recorded the action potential and the force of contraction in the adductor pollicis muscle in response to stimulation of the ulnar nerve. After recording the normal response of the muscle in terms of force of contraction and the motor action potential, the patient was asked to make a maximal voluntary contraction. The tension in the muscle reduced from initial 7 kg to less over a period of 2 minutes. On relaxing the voluntary effort the twitch response to electrical stimulation was negligible but the motor potential was normal. The twitch response also recovered rapidly. When the experiment was repeated with circulation arrest, the muscle became fatigued much earlier but the motor potential was again intact. Thus throughout the whole experiment the motor potential in response to stimulation was normal indicating that the neuromuscular transmission was unimpaired.

Causes of Local Fatigue

The cause of local fatigue lies in the changes that is seen in the muscles itself which was presumably as follows:
- Anoxia
- Depletion of muscle glycogen
- Lack of blood glucose
- Accumulation of metabolites.

Voluntary contraction versus electrical stimulation: Fatigue can be controlled or delayed during voluntary submaximal workout of muscles by varying the particular motor units involved. Prolonged contraction shows increased recruitment of motor units to maintain the same muscle force as fatigue occurs (Berger, 1982). Therefore it can be expected that electrical stimulation of muscles via the motor nerve would lead to relatively rapid muscular fatigue since the fixed set of motor units are being repeatedly stimulated with the fast twitch type II fibers preferentially selected. Currier and Mann, !983 found out that fatigue due to electrical stimulation was greater than that due to isometric voluntary contraction of equal force. Rankin and Stokes 1992 found out that the fatigue caused to the muscle as a result of electrical stimulation was relatively of a longer duration as compared to ones induced as a result of voluntary contraction (speak about the controversy in use of functional electrical stimulation).

General Fatigue

In general fatigue it is not only one muscle or a specific group of muscles but it is the whole body which performs at a sluggish level and demands a period of rest. Unlike in case of local fatigue, here the seat of fatigue lies in the central synapses located in the anterior horn cells or synapses in the brain. The fatigue that sets in a normal person in response to vigorous general body exercises or games is general fatigue. Dexedrine which is an anabolic steroid can delay the onset of general fatigue by acting on the central synapses to lift the performances of sportsman and is an illegal drug.

Common Conditions Causing Fatigue

- *COPD:* There is fatigue of ventilatory muscles which can be either due to weakness, increased load on them, decreased supply of energy to these muscles and due to combination of all these factors.
- *Heart failure:* Generalized fatigue due to poor perfusion of active muscles as a decline of cardiac output.
- *Multiple sclerosis:* One of the most common and usually most disabling symptoms is that of fatigue. It is described as deterioration in performance with continuing effort. It is due to paresis of muscles.
- *Rheumatoid sclerosis:* It is generalized fatigue seen due to progressive weakness and wasting.
- *Myasthenia gravis:* Progressive fatigability is due to an abnormality in the neuromuscular transmission which is mainly due to the defect in the postsynaptic terminal.

FATIGUE ASSESSMENT

The assessment of fatigue can be made by monitoring the changes that occurs during the onset of fatigue. The changes that portrays the onset of fatigue can be systemic as well as or local. Hence the assessment of fatigue should not only involve the local examination but should also assess the systemic changes.

Systemic Assessment

Anaerobic Fatigue

It involves assessment of fatigue during anaerobic power performance when vigorous exercises continues for more than few seconds the short term energy system (Anaerobic glycolysis) generates increasingly more energy for ATP resynthesis than compared to aerobic mechanism.

During short duration high intensity exercises the energy requirement significantly exceeds the energy generated by the hydrogen oxidation in the respiratory chain. Hence anaerobic glycolysis predominates and large quantities of lactate accumulates in active muscles and blood.

Anaerobic fatigue is the percentage decline in the power output during the test. Rate of fatigue is the decline in power in relationship to the peak value.

To test anaerobic fatigue the patient is subjected to anaerobic power performance tests. Performances that substantially activate the short term energy system require maximal exercise for 3 minutes. The various activities that can be given are all out run, bicycle ergometer, shuttle run and weight lifting. The various tests which are used are:

Katch test: The patient was made to perform static cycle with resistance against fywheel which supposedly is to be high load (6 kg for men and 5 kg for women). Duration of the session was 40 seconds. The peak power of pedal cycling represented the patient's anaerobic power. Thus anaerobic fatigue can be found out as the percentage decline in the power output during the test.

Wingate cycle ergometer test: This test is a very popular and latest test available to assess the anaerobic capacity which helps in determining the anaerobic power, anaerobic fatigue and total anaerobic capacity.

Procedure: The subject goes through as session of warm up for about 3 minutes and then begins to pedal the static cycle as fast as he can without resistance. Within 3 seconds the fixed resistance is applied to the flywheel and the subject continues to pedal as fast as he can for 30 seconds. An electrical or mechanical device continuously records flywheel revolutions in 5 seconds interval.

The resistance equals to 0.075 kg per body weight. Thus for a 70 kg person it comes to 5.25 kg.

Test scores

1. *Peak power output (PP):* The highest power out put observed during the first 5 second exercise interval indicates the energy generating capacity of the immediate energy system. PP is expressed in watts and is computed as:

Force × distance

(number of revolutions × distance per revolution)

divided by time in minutes (5 sec = 0.0833 min)

2. *Anaerobic fatigue (AF):* It is the percentage decline in power output during the test. AF represents the total capacity to produce ATP via the immediate and short term energy systems. It is computed as (Highest 5 second PP – lowest 5 second PP) divided by highest 5 second PP × 100.

   Example: If a man weighing 73.3 kg performs wingate test on a Monark cycle ergometer (6.0 m traveled per pedal revolution) with an applied resistance of 5.5 kg (73.3 × 0.075 = 5.49 rounded off to 5.5 kg) , pedal revolution at 5 seconds interval is 12, 10, 8, 7, 6, and 5 (48 total revolutions in 30 seconds).

Peak power output = force × distance divided by time

5.5 kg × (12 × 6) divided by 0.083 min

396 divided by 0.083

= 4753.9 kg –m .min-1 or 776.8 watts (W)

(1 W = 6.12 kg-m.min-1)

Anaerobic fatigue = High power output – low power out put divided by high power out put × 100.

High power output is 776.8 W

Low power output = force × distance divided by time

5.5 × (5 × 6) divided by 0.083

5.5 x 30 / 0.083

= 1980.8 kg-m.min-1 = 323.7 W

Thus, anaerobic fatigue = 776.8 – 323.7 divided by 776.8 ×100 = 58.3%

Measurement of Blood Lactate Levels

The presence of lactate in the muscle and blood indicates the contribution from the anaerobic metabolism to give energy to the work performed. Thus as fatigue is reached the amount of lactate in the blood and muscle is maximum, however the lactate serves as an important substrate in energy storing and energy generating pathways in different tissues. Measurement of lactate in blood can give an idea regarding the extent of fatigue.

Measurement of Aerobic Capacity

The assessment of aerobic system will give information regarding fatigue that occurs due to lack of proper oxygen supply to the exercising structures. This type of aerobic fatigue occurs during a prolonged exercise program when the energy producing sources are the aerobic system. The aerobic capacity of an individual can be measured by calculating his maximal oxygen consumption which is given as VO_2 max. VO_2 max is a measure of the body's capacity of use oxygen. It is usually measured while performing an exercise bout using larger group of muscles like that of swimming, cycling, running, etc. It is the maximum amount of oxygen consumed per minute when the individual has reached maximum effort. It is expressed as milliliters of oxygen per kilogram of body weight per minute (ml/kg per minute). It is dependent on the transport of oxygen, oxygen binding capacity of the blood, cardiac function, oxygen extraction capabilities and muscular oxidative potential. It is given with Fick's equation as:

$$VO_2 \text{ max} = \text{Cardiac output} \times \text{arteriovenous } O_2 \text{ difference}$$
$$= Q \times a - VO_2$$
$$\text{Cardiac output (Q)} = \text{heart rate} \times \text{stroke volume}$$
$$\text{Arteriovenous } O_2 \text{ difference} = \text{arterial } O_2 - \text{venous } O_2$$

Measurement of Energy Expenditure

Energy expenditure can also be determined easily by open circuit portable spirometry and also by telemetry.

In spirometer testing the patient needs to just breath in and out of a mouth piece with a valve. The energy expenditure is computed from the amount of oxygen consumed.

In telemetry or physiologic radio transmission allows the individual to move freely. The heart rate of the individual is transmitted to a graphic printout system. Heart rate is linearly related to the amount of oxygen consumed.

Local Assessment

The local assessment is very helpful in evaluating muscular fatigue and it can be accomplished in different ways. Muscular fatigue results from interruption in the chain of events between the CNS and the muscle fiber. Muscle function deteriorates due to fatigue during any prolonged submaximal exercises. However the recruitment of more and more motor units to perform a specific task of submaximal exercise can delay the onset of fatigue. In a very heavy task activating all the motor units, a decrease in neural activity accompanies fatigue. Thus all those assessment procedures which indicate a fall in the strength or firing ability of the muscle fiber can be used to determine fatigue. The commonly used techniques are as follows:

Electrophysiological Testing

Decremental studies: Muscular fatigue that is produced in certain disorders can be assessed by electrophysiological test. Conditions like Myasthenia gravis, Myasthenic syndrome, McArdle's disease, etc. wherein fatigue is always a cardinal feature often are tested electrophysiologically to assess muscular fatigue. The studies are called as Decremental studies in which on repetitive stimulation of all the muscle fibers, the compound motor potential will show a consistently lesser amplitude indicating the generation of fatigue. The nerve is stimulated by a supramaximal stimulus at slow or faster rate repeatedly so that all the available motor units of the corresponding muscle will fire. Due to abnormality in the neuromuscular transmission it was seen in Myasthenia gravis that with repeated stimulation the corresponding amplitude of the same muscles gradually got lower and lower till the motor potential was no longer produced.

EMG: EMG recording when the patient contracts the muscle voluntary also will show a decrease in the amplitude of the motor unit potential due to the onset of fatigue. Fatigue decreases the force of contraction which contributes to the decrease in the amplitude of the potential.

MMT or manual muscle testing: It is a procedure in which the power generated by the muscle is assessed manually without use of any gadgets. The normal muscle is graded as 5 which indicates normal level of strength. With fatigue the strength generated by the muscle decreases hence the MMT grade of the muscle also comes down.

Infact the procedure of 10 RM testing can also be used to find out whether a specific muscles has entered into a state of fatigue. For instance a normal muscle may have a certain 10 RM under normal circumstances but once fatigue sets it this 10 RM reduces as long as the muscle is in the stage of fatigue. Infact the 10 RM will keep reducing gradually as long as the muscle is continuously exercised. The condition can however come back to normal once a period of rest is given in between.

Endurance testing: Endurance is the ability of the muscle to continuously perform a specific task without a period of rest. To test endurance a muscle is asked to repeat contraction either isometrically or isotonically without any resistance till fatigue occurs. The lesser the repetition indicates more tendency of the muscle to develop fatigue.

SELF-ASSESSING QUESTIONS

Long Essays

a. Describe various methods of assessing fatigue.
b. Describe the method of assessing local fatigue.

Short Essays

a. Define fatigue.
b. What are the causes of fatigue?
c. Different types of fatigue.
d. What is anaerobic fatigue?

Index